Advances in Complex Valvular Disease

Edited by Michael S. Firstenberg and Imran Khan

Published in London, United Kingdom

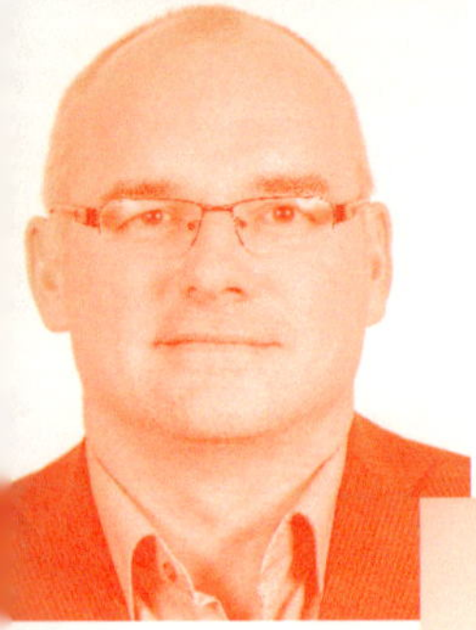
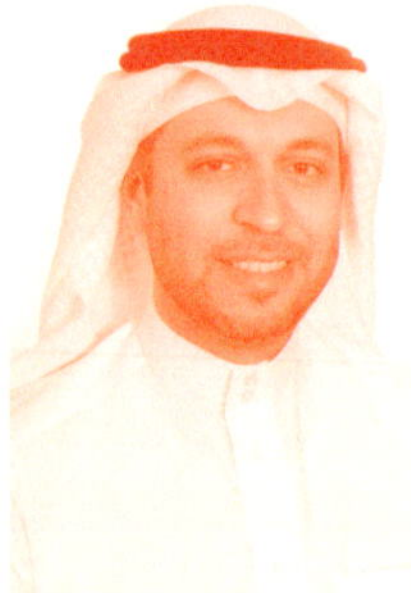
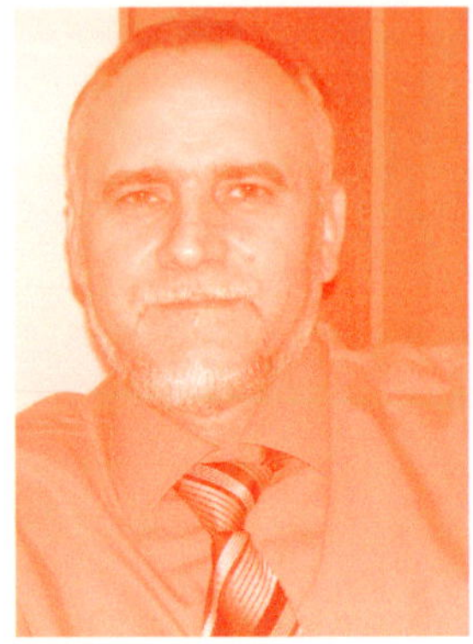
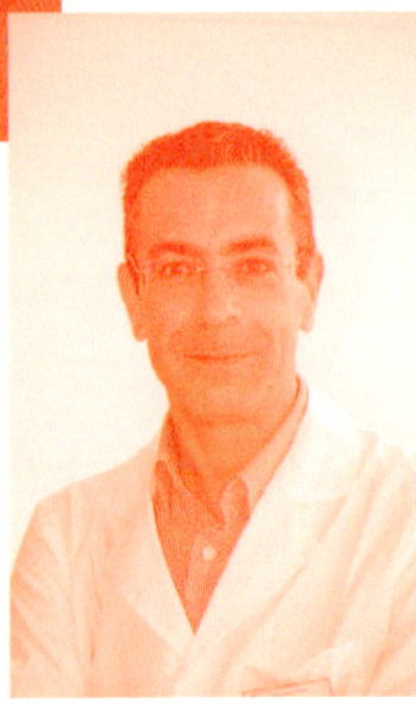
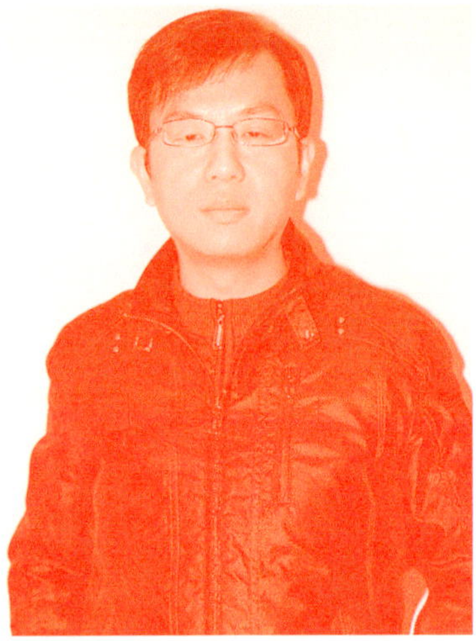
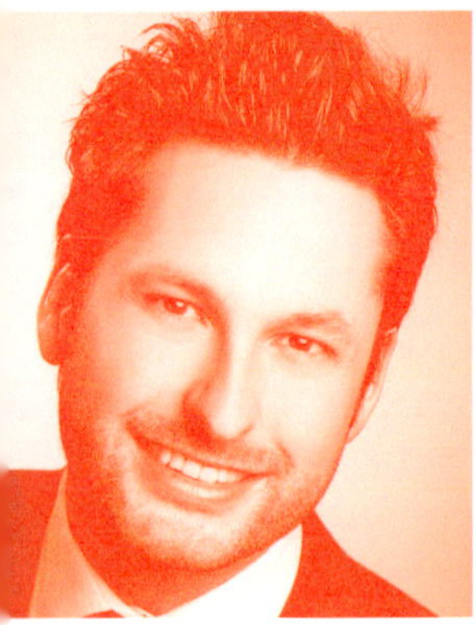
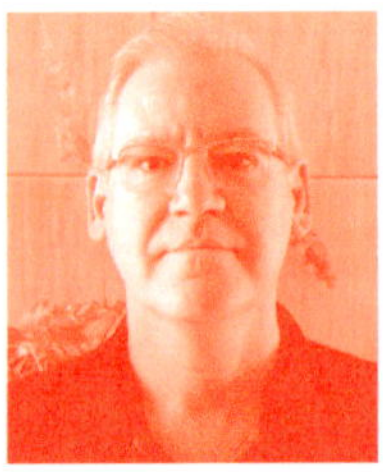

IntechOpen

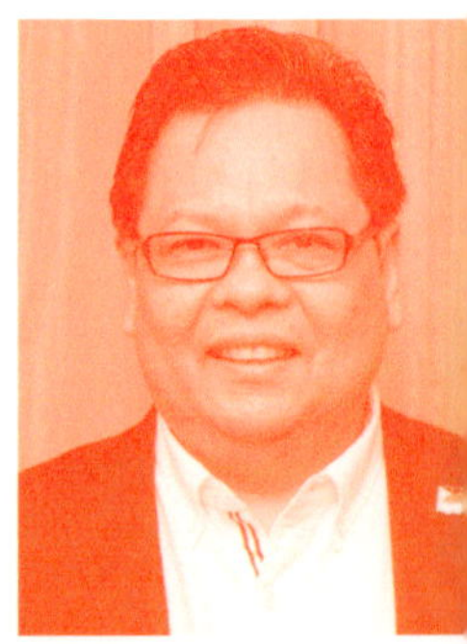
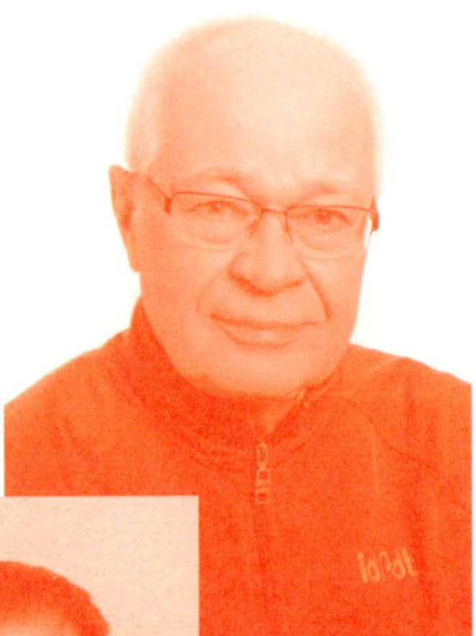
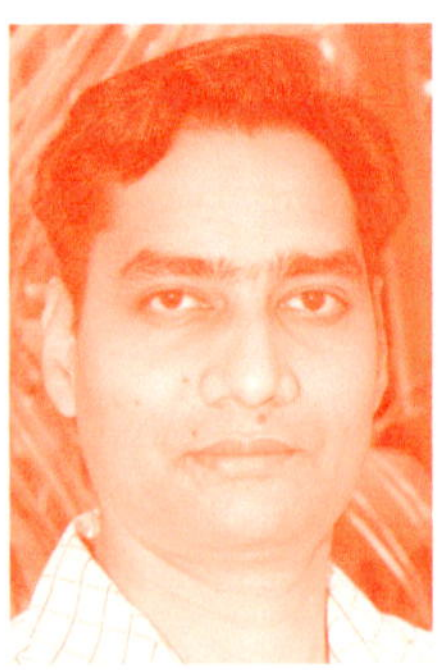
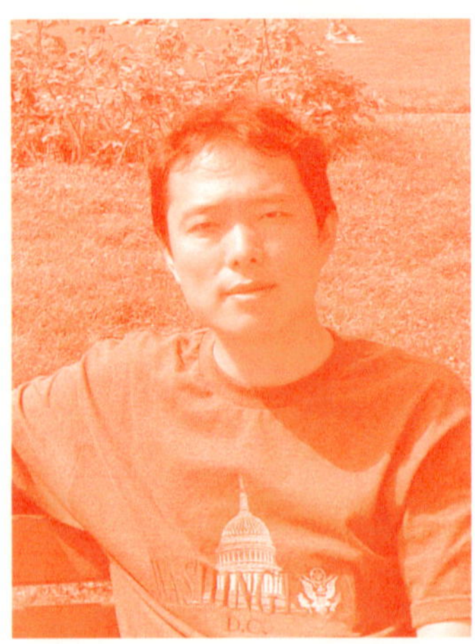
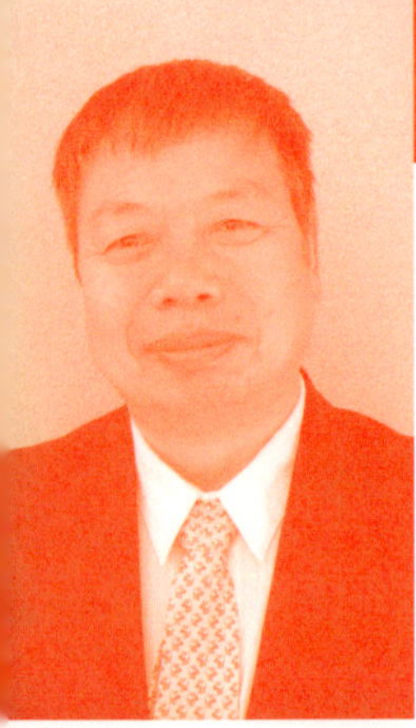
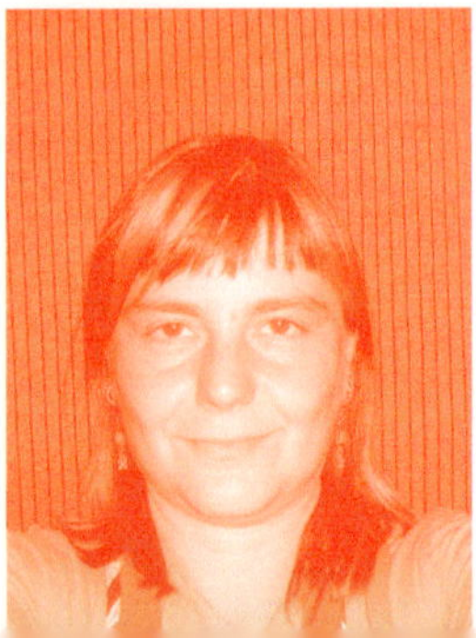

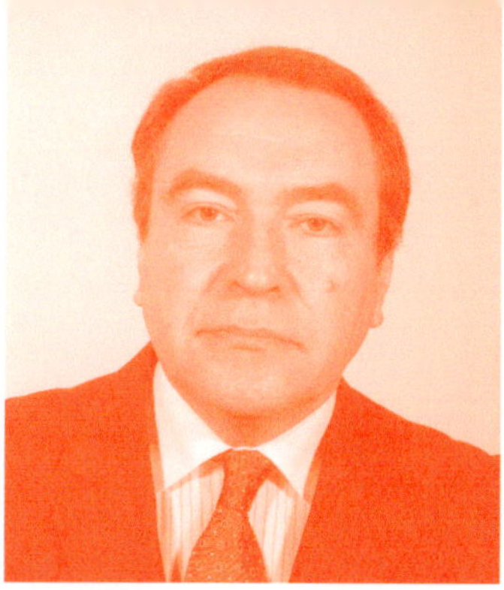
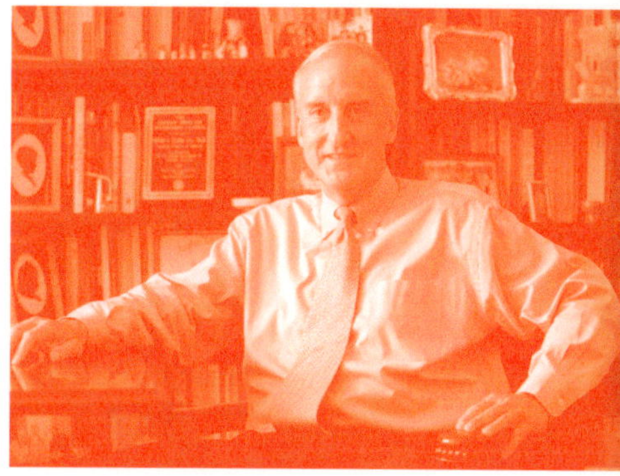
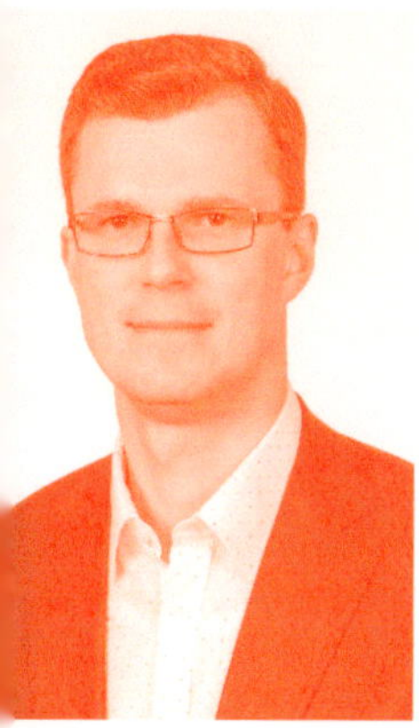
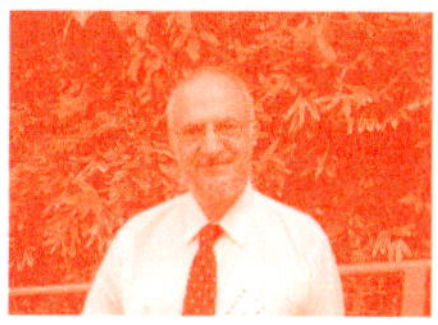
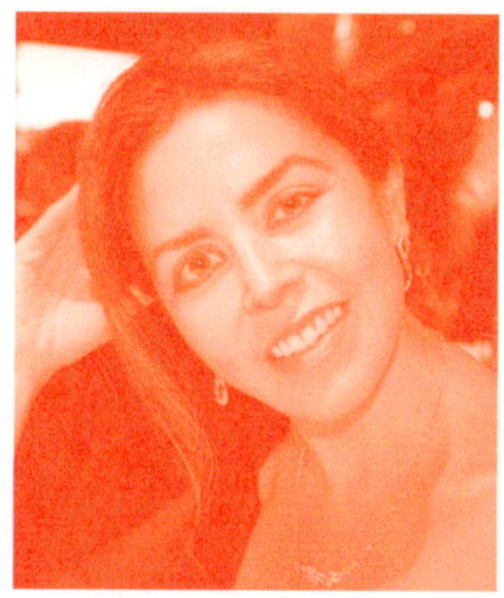

Supporting open minds since 2005

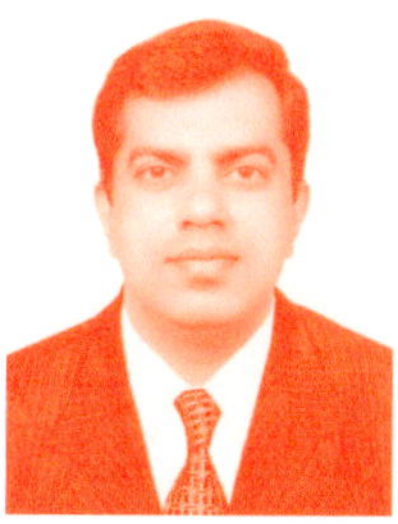
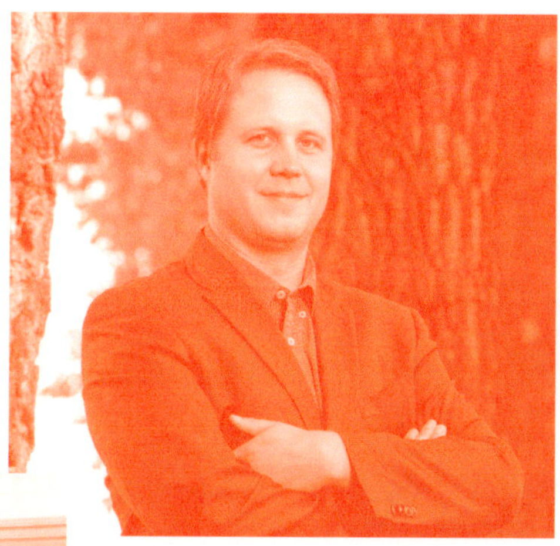
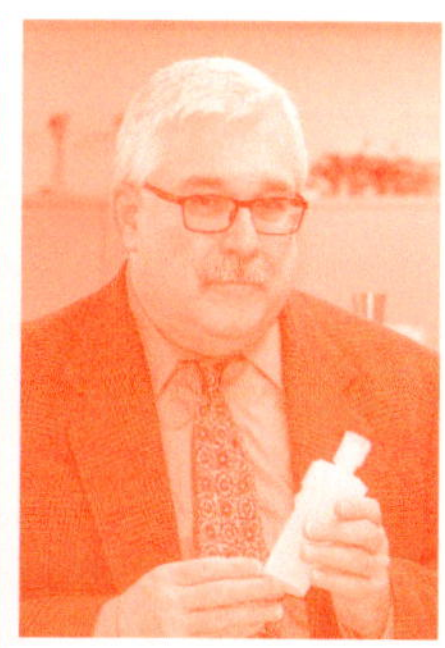
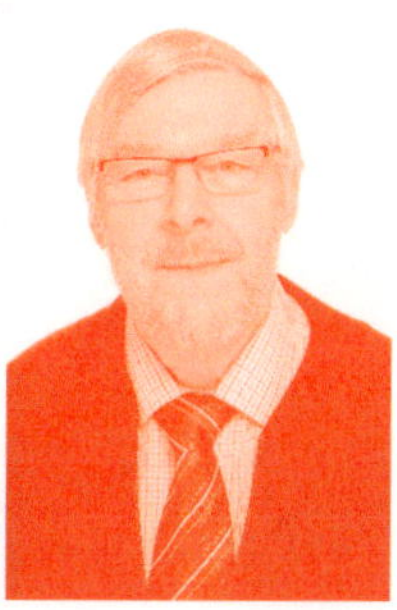
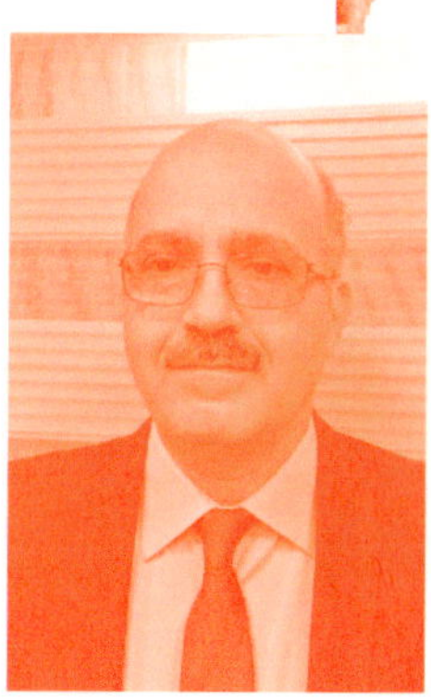
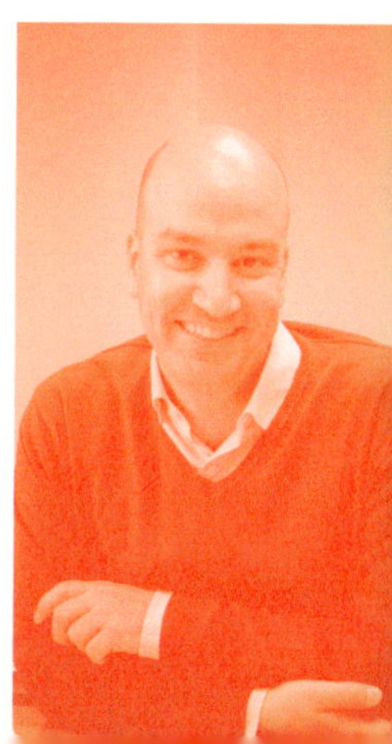
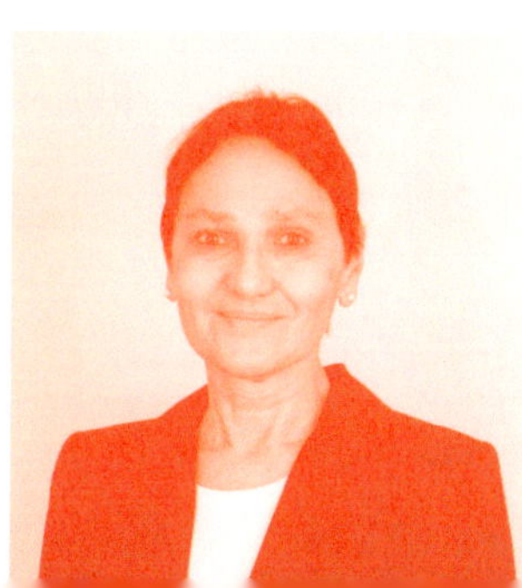

Advances in Complex Valvular Disease
http://dx.doi.org/10.5772/intechopen.87381
Edited by Michael S. Firstenberg and Imran Khan

Contributors
Imran Khan, Julian Smith, Prashant Joshi, Adrian Pick, Adam El-Gamel, Yamile Munoz, Maria Jose Sáenz, Renzo Cifuentes, P. Syamasundar Rao, Ernesto Salcedo, Edward Gill, Haibo Zhang, Michael S. S Firstenberg, Jennifer Hanna, Meng Xu

First published in London, United Kingdom, 2021 by IntechOpen
IntechOpen is the global imprint of INTECHOPEN LIMITED, registered in England and Wales, registration number: 11086078, 5 Princes Gate Court, London, SW7 2QJ, United Kingdom
Printed in Croatia

British Library Cataloguing-in-Publication Data
A catalogue record for this book is available from the British Library

Additional hard and PDF copies can be obtained from orders@intechopen.com

Advances in Complex Valvular Disease
Edited by Michael S. Firstenberg and Imran Khan
p. cm.
Print ISBN 978-1-83968-422-7
Online ISBN 978-1-83968-423-4
eBook (PDF) ISBN 978-1-83968-424-1

For EU product safety concerns:
IN TECH d.o.o., Prolaz Marije Krucifikse Kozulić 3, 51000 Rijeka, Croatia, info@intechopen.com or visit our website at intechopen.com.

Meet the editors

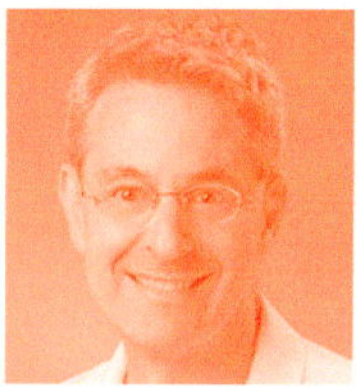

Dr. Firstenberg is a cardiothoracic surgeon and current Director of Research and Special Projects for the William Novick Global Cardiac Alliance. Previously, he was Chief of Cardiothoracic at the Medical Center of Aurora. He attended Case Western Reserve University Medical School, trained in General Surgery at university hospitals in Cleveland and with Cardiothoracic Fellowships at The Ohio State University and The Cleveland Clinic. He is active in numerous medical societies and a Founding Fellow and President-elect of the American College of Academic International Medicine. He has lectured extensively worldwide and authored over 200 peer-reviewed manuscripts, abstracts, and book chapters. He has edited numerous textbooks ranging from Medical Leadership, Patient Safety, and Extra-corporeal Membrane Oxygenation.

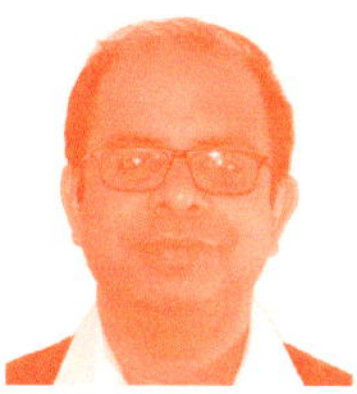

Dr. Imran Khan is currently working as a Cardiothoracic Surgery Registrar in the Department of Cardio-thoracic Surgery, Royal North Shore Hospital, Sydney. Prior to this, he was working as a Fellow in Cardiothoracic Surgery at Monash Medical Centre, Clayton with Prof Julian Smith and his team. Before coming to Australia, he was working as an Associate Consultant in the Department of Cardiac Surgery at Medanta Hospital, Gurgaon, India. It is a tertiary care 1200-bed hospital. The department of Cardiac Surgery performs around 3000 cases per year. He completed his training in Cardiac Vascular & Thoracic Surgery (M.Ch.) from the Post Graduate Institute of Medical & Research (P.GI.M.E.R.), Chandigarh, India. His research project was on the "Relation of histology and ultra-structure of left atrium in Mitral valve disease with Atrial Fibrillation: Correlation with left atrium size and cardioversion". He with Dr. Naresh Trehan (Chief Cardiac Surgeon) at Medanta Hospital, Gurgaon. There he was exposed to almost the entire spectrum of adult cardiac surgery. Apart from taking active participation in the operating room, he was actively involved in pre-operative and post-operative care of patients. I was also the Principal Investigator of the research project 'Study to determine the index of completeness of revascularization and incidence of stroke in off-pump and on-pump coronary artery bypass grafting'. Recently, he presented papers in EACTS, AATS, and IACTS conferences. His 2 chapters on 'Current and future management strategies of type A Aortic dissection' and 'Minimally Invasive Right Anterior Mini-Thoracotomy Aortic Valve Replacement' have been published in cardiac surgery books in the last 2 years. His application for specialist assessment with the Royal Australasian College of Surgeons has been found to be comparable, and he will be taking further training before sitting for his FRACS exam. He has been exposed to a good number of elective and emergent adult cardiac and aortic cases including redo cases back in India and in Australia. Now, he has a keen interest to widen his skill-set by working in a unit specializing in heart and lung transplant and heart failure management strategies and minimally invasive cardiac surgery.

Contents

Preface

The assessment and management of complex valve disease have changed substantially over the past 10 years. This evolution has been fueled by simultaneous advances in diagnostic and therapeutic innovations that have offered renewed hope for one of the most common forms of heart disease in advanced societies. The goals of this volume are to highlight some of the state-of-the-art advances in valve management and to help put it into a context that is scientifically accessible to readers, students, healthcare providers, and maybe even patients and their families at all levels of understanding. While this text is by no means meant to be a definitive review of all of the revolutionary advances in aortic valve disease – as such an effort would be a tremendous undertaking spanning extensive volumes and most likely be out-of-date shortly after publication due to such rapid advances in the field – it is meant to be a foundation for building on a further understanding of where we have been, where we are, and hopefully where we are going.

The focus of this text can be divided into several key areas. First and foremost is a basic review of the latest developments in understanding aortic valve pathology. This is then followed by the outlining of some of the advanced diagnostic imaging tools to better understand the progression and natural history of aortic valve pathology. Separate chapters on different types of valve pathology – such as the association with aortic dissections and relationships to some of the complex challenges associated with univentricular congenital palliative procedures – are also reviewed. In addition, the revolution of transcatheter aortic valve therapies – again, a topic that is one of the largest areas of global students – is also discussed in the context of current options for the management of stenotic and regurgitant valves.

Many of the topics of this volume reflect areas that are constantly evolving and hopefully each chapter can serve as a basic foundation to encourage the reader to explore the references and help direct them towards the latest advances that are being discovered almost daily.

As the Editor, I wanted to thank all of the authors for the contributions to this project and to the readers for allowing all of us to help kindle a larger interest in such a complex and dynamic topic.

Michael S. Firstenberg
The Medical Center of Aurora,
United States of America

Imran Khan
Monash Medical Centre,
Australia

Section 1

Aortic Valve Disease

Chapter 1

Introductory Chapter: The Evolution of Complex Valve Pathology - The Surgeon's Perspective

Michael S. Firstenberg and Jennifer Hanna

1. Introduction

The management of aortic valve disease has undergone a dramatic transformation over the past 10 years. Without a doubt there has been significant developments in the diagnostic and management tools available to assess patients with aortic valve pathology. In addition to these tools are better and safer surgical techniques, especially with regards to anesthesia, myocardial protection, and peri-operative care, as well as the means in which patients can be risk-assessed to help guide decision-making. However, despite these advances, patients presenting with significant valvular disease are getting older and often will have substantial and more complex co-morbidities that place them at significant risk for challenging short- and long-term adverse outcomes. The goal of this text is to illustrate some of the challenges and controversies, with an emphasis on a surgical perspective, regarding the diagnosis and management of one of the most common forms of degenerative valve disease – aortic stenosis. While, by no means, is this a comprehensive review, it does provide a foundation and potential paradigm for how we evaluate, manage, and study valve disease both at a patient as well as a population level.

2. Background

Aortic stenosis is the most prevalent form of native valvular disease. Significant stenosis, as determined by the gradients across the valve and estimated orifice areas, are encountered in up to 2% of the population over 65 years old, 3% in those over 75 years old and 4% over 85 years old. Furthermore, over 100,000 people in the United States alone are diagnosed with severe aortic stenosis each year. Historically, the management of severe and critical aortic stenosis, especially in the context of symptoms such as chest pain, syncope, and shortness of breath, has focused on surgical intervention. However, the risks increase substantially with patients age and comorbidities [1].

Typically, severe or critical stenosis is manifested with the onset of symptoms such as shortness of breath. However, when patients start developing heart failure, chest pain, or syncope, their prognosis becomes worse than many cancers, including breast and colon. In fact, without intervention, the estimated survival in this population is less than 50% at two years [2].

3. Treatment options

It has been well established that the mortality difference between symptomatic aortic stenosis patients treated with surgery and those treated medically is one of the most striking mortality differences in all of medicine. In fact, it is argued that it is unethical to withhold therapy in symptomatic patients regardless of approach unless there are compelling contraindications. The percent survival of critical aortic stenosis patients is less than 20% at two years compared to a greater than 85% 4- to 5-year survival in those undergoing surgery [3]. A variety of tools have been developed over the years regarding risk assessment for surgery to aid in decision-making. One of the most commonly used is the Society of Thoracic Surgeons predicted risk of mortality calculator [4, 5]. Additional variables include a formal assessment of patient frailty, existing comorbidities and major organ system dysfunction, and technical or anatomical aspects of the procedure that may increase perioperative risks. Putting all of these variables together allows patients to be stratified as low, intermediate, high, and prohibitive risk. These tools are then used to help patients participate in shared decision-making regarding management options as guided by a Heart Team of cardiovascular specialists [6]. Historically, the options for treatment focused on surgery with a variety of biologic and mechanical valve choices – each with advantages and disadvantages, with trade-offs being either durability or the need for lifelong anticoagulation. The development over the past 10 to 15 years of catheter-based options, specifically transaortic valve replacement (TAVR) has resulted in a dramatic increase in therapies offered to patients who otherwise were prohibitive risk [7, 8]. Recent data has allowed for catheter-based therapies to be offered to lower risk populations [9]. However, despite the appeal of catheter-based therapies over conventional open-heart surgery, there are still many questions that need to be answered with regards to durability, paravalvular leaks, need for permanent pacemaker implantation, and the growing concerns surrounding both short- and long-term complications that are only slowly being definitively reported. Nevertheless, despite the evolving data and significant amount of industry-driven support stimulating the excitement over transcatheter therapies, combined with the significant costs associated with these based therapies, there are still concerns that surgery might still be the preferred approach for certain patients.

Some of the initial multi-center randomized trials that focused on high and extreme risk patients demonstrated a survival advantage which led to a considerable amount of enthusiasm regarding the potential for catheter-based valves as a viable option for patients who would otherwise die of complications related to their critical aortic stenosis. Following regulatory approval of these devices, additional studies in intermediate and lower risk patients were undertaken. While the selection criteria for intermediate risk patients was based upon their predicted risk of mortality, other significant comorbidities and baseline characteristics were considered in the decision-making. Again, despite the appeal of non-surgical options, the early data in the intermediate risk patient population demonstrated similar all-cause mortality and risk of disabling stroke of around 13 to 14% at two years [10]. These results suggested that catheter-based therapies were non-inferior to surgical approaches, and despite the similarities in outcomes, these findings have often been cited to imply that a non-surgical approach may be preferred by the patients and are even potentially superior with regards to both short- and long-term outcomes when compared to conventional surgery [11]. In fact, while surgery was associated with a period of recovery that impacted formal quality of life assessments, by six months, the objective assessment of quality of life was similar in the surgical and catheter-based patients. In addition, similar short- and long-term mortality and stroke risks were seen in low, intermediate, and higher risk patients, again illustrating that both approaches were similar with regards to patient outcomes. Nevertheless, there has been a significant appeal, for a variety of reasons, for trans-catheter therapies, and numerous studies have been undertaken to define which patient characteristics and comorbidities might be better suited for one therapy over the other. A review of 9500 intermediate risk patients enrolled in multiple studies showed no significant benefit of one therapy over another at one year [12]. Similar reviews were also performed in lower risk patients. Specifically looking at the mortality at two years in almost 3500 patients, there was no benefit to a trans-catheter approach over surgery, further emphasizing the concept of non-inferior outcomes [13]. In this meta-analysis, there were also similar outcomes with regards to procedure-related stroke. However, there was evidence of a potential 2-year survival advantage for patients undergoing surgery. This survival advantage was also seen in a meta-analysis of intermediate risk patients enrolled in 14 studies consisting of almost 4200 patients. All told, at three years, there appeared to be a significant survival advantage for the intermediate risk patients undergoing surgical aortic valve replacement when compared to trans-catheter therapies [14]. Despite these concerns regarding the long-term outcomes in patients undergoing catheter-based therapies, there have been several randomized multi-center studies exploring their potential role in lower risk patients. The early data has suggested non-inferior outcomes, although some suggest a potential small survival advantage in those undergoing catheter-based therapies with specific types of valves. However, these trials have been heavily criticized. For example, in the PARTNER-3 trial, there was some concern that, despite enrolling low risk patients only, some of the comorbidities and surgical procedures required for these patients implied an inherently much higher risk profile [15]. Furthermore, there was concern that many patients were excluded based upon anatomical considerations, and patient selection might have played a substantial role in reported outcomes favoring catheter-based therapies [16]. Other low risk trials validated some of the short-term outcome experiences that contributed to regulatory approval with low-risk patients. A fundamental consideration is that low risk is not synonymous with younger patients, and given some of the evolving concerns surrounding intermediate- and long-term survival differences, there are still substantial concerns about offering catheter-based therapies to patients who have a predicted life expectancy beyond several years. Unfortunately, this has not attenuated the astronomical growth of catheter-based therapies at the expense of surgery in a patient population that still, based upon best available evidence, might still benefit from a surgical approach.

The selection bias and concerns of the low-risk trials for TAVR have prompted investigators to report some of the real-world outcomes in similar patients. For example, registry data out of Israel looking at very low risk and low risk patients demonstrated a 10 to 15% two-year mortality, respectively [17]. These outcomes were substantially worse than similar two-year survival rates reported in contemporary surgical studies in which the reported mortality was almost half of those reported in similar TAVR patients [18]. It is unclear if patients are aware of the substantial risks of these procedures when they are making decisions or are being consented.

Clearly, there is still much to learn with regards to the risks, benefits, and patient selection for specific therapies used to treat aortic stenosis. Furthermore, as experiences evolve, especially with the rapid proliferation of transcatheter therapies, there are still many challenges and unanswered questions.

4. Evolving controversies

4.1 Stroke

There is a common misconception that trans-catheter therapies are inherently associated with fewer strokes. This is an observation that has not been demonstrated in many of the high-profile studies. Furthermore, there are growing concerns that the neurologic events that patients experience after trans-catheter therapies occur after the index hospitalization in which the procedure is performed. For example, one study exploring a Medicare database of over 44,000 patients suggested an 86% greater risk of ischemic stroke and a six-fold increase risk of hemorrhagic stroke after trans-catheter therapies when compared to conventional surgery, with many of the events occurring in subsequent readmissions to the hospital within the first year [19]. In fact, the 90-day readmission rate for neurologic events after TAVR was substantially higher than many other cardiac and non-cardiac procedures, including left ventricular assist device placement, cardiac catheterization, surgical aortic valve replacement, and coronary artery bypass procedures [20]. Clearly, the risk of neurologic events after catheter-based valvular interventions requires further objective review.

Such concerns have resulted in a substantial increase in the development and utilization of cerebral protection devices during TAVR. Despite the inherent appeal and considerable cost associated with these protection devices, definitive data demonstrating a clinical improvement and reduction in neurologic events is still lacking [21, 22]. Nevertheless, this is an area of tremendous research and development [23, 24].

4.2 Pacemaker rates

There is no doubt, as demonstrated in almost every major study of TAVR, that this procedure is associated with a much greater risk for needing a permanent pacemaker when compared to conventional surgery. While conduction abnormalities are not uncommon after valve surgery, there is growing concern that the need for a pacemaker after TAVR is neither trivial nor benign. Some large-scale studies suggest a four-fold increase in the need for permanent pacemaker after TAVR [25]. While the long-term consequences of needing a pacemaker are still unclear, especially since the short and long-term natural history of conduction problems after valve replacement is variable, there is evidence to suggest that the need for a pacemaker is associated with worse long-term survival in these patients [26]. Considering the growing emphasis on early discharge and the concern that some of the conduction abnormalities might be physiologically significant and not present until after the index hospitalization, the consequences of such events is still unclear [27].

4.3 Paravalvular leaks

Unlike surgical valve replacement in which the existing stenotic calcified valve is physically removed, TAVR inserts and expands against the existing valve. This fundamental difference in the two procedures can explain why TAVR is still associated with a significantly higher rate of paravalvular leaks – especially in those with eccentric valve pathology or bicuspid valves [28]. Again, the long-term significance of paravalvular leaks is incompletely defined, but without a doubt, those patients with at least moderate leaks have a much worse survival at 2 years than those with mild or less leaks. The PARTNER 2 study, as previously discussed above, demonstrated a 34% risk of mortality in patients with moderate to severe paravalvular leaks, when compared to the 13-14% risk in those with none, trace, or mild leaks [29]

4.4 Durability and cost

Durability and cost remain a considerable concern regarding catheter-based therapies. Although costs vary significantly depending on the intrinsic structure of a health-care system, conflicting evidence regarding the short- and long-term costs of different types of therapy for valvular disease exists. Without a doubt, a surgical valve is substantially less expensive than a catheter-based valve, but the overall costs of the hospitalization and short-term rehabilitation needs might be more. However, factoring in the needs for pacemakers, stroke management, and concomitant coronary disease, there is growing concern surrounding the real-world costs for catheter-based therapies – especially as an increasing number of patients with advanced comorbidities, age, and poor functional status are being treated prior to dying [30, 31].

4.5 Coronary artery interventions

Especially with patients who are older and have multiple comorbidities, the incidence of coronary artery disease further challenges clinical decision-making. Again, despite the appeal of catheter-based solutions to treat both obstructive coronary disease and aortic valve pathology, definitive data directing one therapeutic option over another is lacking. In fact, many of the initial studies exploring the outcomes of one approach over another specifically excluded concomitant coronary procedures or those patients with significant obstructive disease. Nevertheless, criticism of some of the more recent low risk trials is that the surgical patients had a much higher intrinsic risk profile because of the need for concomitant coronary revascularization. In addition, structural characteristics of artificial valves also raises concerns regarding difficulties in coronary access in patients with previous valve replacements (both surgical and TAVR) and further suggests the importance of complete revascularization at the time of definitive valve therapies. As mentioned, many studies specifically excluded patients with combined aortic stenosis and coronary artery disease, and current guidelines tend to favor surgery considering the limitations of the data [32, 33]. Preliminary data also suggests that patients undergoing coronary stenting prior to TAVR may have worse outcomes and increased need for re-interventions due to major adverse cardiac and cerebrovascular events [34, 35].

4.6 Repeat interventions

The area of aortic valve disease that probably is the most supportive of trans-catheter therapies is in patients that have had previous valve replacement, either with a previous surgical valve or a trans-catheter valve. Many patients underwent surgical replacement with a biologic valve, despite established guidelines and a potential survival advantage advocating the use of a mechanical valve under the promise that their next intervention would be a trans-catheter valve [36, 37]. While the appeal of this approach is undeniable and logical, the practical applications are still under considerable study. Conflicting data regarding the best approach for the management of a failing biologic valve is substantial. Even though repeat surgery is not without risks, many experienced centers can offer re-operative surgery with a risk profile similar to first-time valve replacement. Furthermore, there are concerns surrounding a reduction in the effective orifice areas and the risk for patient-prosthesis mismatch after placement of a TAVR inside of a previous surgical or trans-catheter valve.

4.7 Choice of valves

In the surgical era, the choice of valves consisted of tissue valves and mechanical valves. Mechanical valves required life-long anticoagulation and this was often unappealing to patients, despite studies demonstrating a long-term survival advantage. Tissue valves did not require long-term anticoagulation, but were associated with structural degeneration and the need for repeat interventions – often at significant risk as outlined above. Many different types of biologic valves exist – bovine, porcine, homographs, stentless, etc – and there is extensive literature generated over decades of experience regarding the advantages and disadvantages of each valve type. Much of the decision-making regarding the initial valve choice is now under debate with the development of catheter-based therapies that can be used for failing biologic valves. Since the concept (as mentioned above) of "valve-in-a-valve" has altered the natural history of the long-term outcomes associated with biologic valves, there is growing interest in their use in younger patients and in the use of those prosthetic valves with structural characteristics that might lend themselves to a more favorable scaffolding for future re-interventions. Concepts surrounding strut design and annular cracking (or fracking) to increase the annular size to allow for larger replacement valves are rapidly evolving areas of study [38]. Likewise, the choice of transcatheter valve design – annular, supra-annular, self- vs balloon-expanding -- and tissue characteristics are also areas of extensive clinical research and debate.

4.8 Indications for intervention

The guidelines for intervention on critical aortic stenosis have also been evolving to reflect the developments in therapy options. However, there is growing evidence to suggest that adverse, and potentially irreversible, structural changes in the myocardium occur prior to the development of symptoms. Even patients with very advanced disease can have minimal symptoms, and much research is being directed towards, as illustrated by the chapter on strain-rate assessment of valvular disease, more objective tools to assess the pathophysiologic consequences of valvular pathology. Tools such as cardiac magnetic resonance imaging, strain-rate, and stress-echocardiography are becoming more commonly used in complex clinical cases to help direct management decisions.

4.9 Other areas of debate

The list of potential controversial topics in the diagnosis and management of valvular disease is extensive and beyond the scope of a simple chapter or even text. Such areas only illustrate the complexity of valve disease and, especially in the context of newer options for therapy, how there are great opportunities to re-explore the options patients have for aortic valve interventions. Even the methods we have to guide therapies – such as the development of Heart Teams (similar to cancer tumor boards in which each patient's clinical characteristics and pathologies are reviewed to make an optimal decision based upon expertise and best available data) and "shared decision making" (a concept in which the patient plays a substantial role in deciding how they want to be treated after weighing the pros/cons of the options as presented to them) – continue to evolve [39].

Other areas that only scratch the surface regarding the management of valve disease include:

- Endocarditis
  - Native vs prosthetic valve
  - Early vs late surgical vs medical management
  - Re-operative options in the setting of substance abuse
  - Indications for left-sided vs right-sided valves
- Aortic insufficiency
  - Timing of surgery
  - Role of catheter-based therapy
- Bicuspid valve disease
- Associated ascending aortic aneurysms and pathology
- Impact of previous cardiac surgery
- Special patient populations
  - End-stage renal disease – i.e. dialysis
  - Morbid obesity
  - Small/large aortic roots
  - Complex co-morbidities
  - "Younger" patients
  - Women of child-bearing age
  - Impact of other co-morbidities
    1. Frailty
    2. End-stage pathologies – i.e. liver, lung, cancers
    3. Age
- Role of anticoagulation/anti-platelet agents
  - Impact on short-term risk for stroke
  - Risk for tissue or valve degeneration/thickening

- Interventions in asymptomatic patients
- Impact of and options for concomitant cardiac pathologies
    - Atrial fibrillation
    - Obstructive coronary artery disease
    - Other valvular pathologies
        1. Mitral, tricuspid
    - Aortic aneurysms
- Evolving repair technologies
- Prosthetic tissue and structural options
    - Bovine vs porcine vs non-biologic
    - Anti-calcification treatments
    - Stented vs non-stented
    - Stent material

5. Conclusions

The list of topics that can be reviewed is endless, clearly beyond the scope of a single text, and only serves to illustrates the importance of having a solid foundation in the existing literature, guidelines, and technologies as we move forward with regards to how we objectively assess and manage patient with aortic valve pathology. While patient preferences clearly should have a role, it is imperative that patients and their families be provided with accurate and objective data that take their personal characteristics into consideration so that their decisions can be properly guided with the goal of optimizing their opportunities for an ideal short- and long-term outcome. Hopefully, texts such as this along with multidisciplinary Heart Teams can help improve these short- and long-term outcomes in terms of quality and quantity of life for those patients with significant valvular pathology.

Conflict of interest

Dr Firstenberg serves as a heart valve repair and replacement educational consultant for Medtronic plc. Dr Hanna reports no conflicts of interest or relevant disclosures in the context of the material presented in this chapter.

Author details

Michael S. Firstenberg[1]* and Jennifer Hanna[2]

1 Research and Special Projects: William Novick Global Cardiac Alliance, Memphis, TN, US

2 Department of Cardiothoracic and Vascular Surgery, The Medical Center of Aurora, Aurora, CO, US

*Address all correspondence to: msfirst@gmail.com; michael.firstenberg@cardiac-alliance.org

References

[1] Iung B, Baron G, Butchart EG, Delahaye F. Gohlke-Brwolf C, Levang OW, Tornos P, Vanoverschelde JL, Vermeer F, Boersma E, Ravaud P, Alec Vahanian. A prospective survey of patients with valvular heart disease in Europe: The Euro Heart Survey on Valvular Heart Disease. Eu Heart J. 2003;24:1231-43.

[2] Lester SJ, Heilbron B, Gin K, Dodek A, Jue J. The natural history and rate of progression of aortic stenosis. Chest. 1998 Apr 1;113(4):1109-14.

[3] Perera S, Wijesinghe N, Ly E, Devlin G, Pasupati S. Outcomes of patients with untreated severe aortic stenosis in real-world practice. NZ Med J. 2011 Nov 4;124(1345):40-8.

[4] Thourani VH, Suri RM, Gunter RL, Sheng S, O'Brien SM, Ailawadi G, Szeto WY, Dewey TM, Guyton RA, Bavaria JE, Babaliaros V. Contemporary real-world outcomes of surgical aortic valve replacement in 141,905 low-risk, intermediate-risk, and high-risk patients. The Annals of thoracic surgery. 2015 Jan 1;99(1):55-61.

[5] http://riskcalc.sts.org/stswebriskcalc/calculate

[6] Holmes DR, Rich JB, Zoghbi WA, Mack MJ. The heart team of cardiovascular care. Journal of the American College of Cardiology. 2013 Mar 5;61(9):903-7.

[7] Mack MJ, Leon MB, Smith CR, Miller DC, Moses JW, Tuzcu EM, Webb JG, Douglas PS, Anderson WN, Blackstone EH, Kodali SK. 5-year outcomes of transcatheter aortic valve replacement or surgical aortic valve replacement for high surgical risk patients with aortic stenosis (PARTNER 1): a randomised controlled trial. The Lancet. 2015 Jun 20;385(9986):2477-84.

[8] Gleason TG, Reardon MJ, Popma JJ, Deeb GM, Yakubov SJ, Lee JS, Kleiman NS, Chetcuti S, Hermiller JB, Heiser J, Merhi W. 5-Year outcomes of self-expanding transcatheter versus surgical aortic valve replacement in high-risk patients. Journal of the American College of Cardiology. 2018 Dec 4;72(22):2687-96.

[9] Popma JJ, Deeb GM, Yakubov SJ, Mumtaz M, Gada H, O'Hair D, Bajwa T, Heiser JC, Merhi W, Kleiman NS, Askew J. Transcatheter aortic-valve replacement with a self-expanding valve in low-risk patients. New England Journal of Medicine. 2019 May 2;380(18):1706-15.

[10] Reardon MJ, Van Mieghem NM, Popma JJ, Kleiman NS, Søndergaard L, Mumtaz M, Adams DH, Deeb GM, Maini B, Gada H, Chetcuti S. Surgical or transcatheter aortic-valve replacement in intermediate-risk patients. New England Journal of Medicine. 2017 Apr 6;376(14):1321-31.

[11] Søndergaard L, Popma JJ, Reardon MJ, Van Mieghem NM, Deeb GM, Kodali S, George I, Williams MR, Yakubov SJ, Kappetein AP, Serruys PW. Comparison of a complete percutaneous versus surgical approach to aortic valve replacement and revascularization in patients at intermediate surgical risk: results from the randomized SURTAVI trial. Circulation. 2019 Oct 15;140(16):1296-305.

[12] Brennan JM, Thomas L, Cohen DJ, Shahian D, Wang A, Mack MJ, Holmes DR, Edwards FH, Frankel NZ, Baron SJ, Carroll J. Transcatheter versus surgical aortic valve replacement: propensity-matched comparison. Journal of the American College of Cardiology. 2017 Jul 25;70(4):439-50.

[13] Witberg G, Lador A, Yahav D, Kornowski R. Transcatheter versus

surgical aortic valve replacement in patients at low surgical risk: a meta-analysis of randomized trials and propensity score matched observational studies. Catheterization and Cardiovascular Interventions. 2018 Aug 1;92(2):408-16.

[14] Takagi H, Mitta S, Ando T, ALICE (All-Literature Investigation of Cardiovascular Evidence) group. Long-term survival after transcatheter versus surgical aortic valve replacement for aortic stenosis: A meta-analysis of observational comparative studies with a propensity-score analysis. Catheterization and Cardiovascular Interventions. 2018 Aug 1;92(2):419-30.

[15] Mack MJ, Leon MB, Thourani VH, Makkar R, Kodali SK, Russo M, Kapadia SR, Malaisrie SC, Cohen DJ, Pibarot P, Leipsic J. Transcatheter aortic-valve replacement with a balloon-expandable valve in low-risk patients. New England Journal of Medicine. 2019 May 2;380(18):1695-705.

[16] Shahim B, Malaisrie SC, George I, Thourani V, Russo M, Biviano A, Mack M, Brown DL, Babaliaros V, Guyton R, Kodali S. TCT CONNECT-468 Postoperative Atrial Fibrillation or Flutter Following Transcatheter or Surgical Aortic Valve Replacement for Severe Aortic Stenosis in Patients at Low Surgical Risk: An Analysis From the PARTNER 3 Trial. Journal of the American College of Cardiology. 2020 Oct 27;76(17 Supplement S):B200-.

[17] Finkelstein A, Rozenbaum Z, Halkin A, Banai S, Bazan S, Barbash I, Segev A, Fefer P, Maor E, Danenberg H, Planner D. Outcomes of transcatheter aortic valve implantation in patients with low versus intermediate to high surgical risk. The American journal of cardiology. 2019 Feb 15;123(4):644-9.

[18] Klautz RJ, Kappetein AP, Lange R, Dagenais F, Labrousse L, Bapat V, Moront M, Misfeld M, Zeng C, Sabik III JF, PERIGON Investigators. Safety, effectiveness and haemodynamic performance of a new stented aortic valve bioprosthesis. European Journal of Cardio-Thoracic Surgery. 2017 Sep 1;52(3):425-31.

[19] Stein L, Thaler A, Liang JW, Tuhrim S, Dhamoon AS, Dhamoon MS. Intermediate-Term Risk of Stroke Following Cardiac Procedures in a Nationally Representative Data Set. Journal of the American Heart Association. 2017 Dec 2;6(12):e006900.

[20] Stein LK, Thaler A, Liang JW, Tuhrim S, Dhamoon AS, Dhamoon MS. Intermediate Risk of Stroke Following Cardiac Procedures in a Nationally Representative Dataset. InANNALS OF NEUROLOGY 2017 Oct 1 (Vol. 82, pp. S49-S49). 111 RIVER ST, HOBOKEN 07030-5774, NJ USA: WILEY.

[21] Giustino G, Sorrentino S, Mehran R, Faggioni M, Dangas G. Cerebral embolic protection during TAVR: a clinical event meta-analysis. Journal of the American College of Cardiology. 2017 Jan 31;69(4):465-6.

[22] Ndunda PM, Vindhyal MR, Muutu TM, Fanari Z. Clinical outcomes of sentinel cerebral protection system use during transcatheter aortic valve replacement: a systematic review and meta-analysis. Cardiovascular Revascularization Medicine. 2020 Jun 1;21(6):717-22.

[23] Haussig S, Mangner N, Dwyer MG, Lehmkuhl L, Lücke C, Woitek F, Holzhey DM, Mohr FW, Gutberlet M, Zivadinov R, Schuler G. Effect of a cerebral protection device on brain lesions following transcatheter aortic valve implantation in patients with severe aortic stenosis: the CLEAN-TAVI randomized clinical trial. Jama. 2016 Aug 9;316(6):592-601.

[24] Alkhouli M, Alqahtani F, Harris AH, Hohmann SF, Rihal CS. Early Experience With Cerebral Embolic Protection During Transcatheter Aortic Valve Replacement in the United States. JAMA internal medicine. 2020 May 1;180(5):783-4.

[25] Subramani S, Arora L, Krishnan S, Hanada S, Sharma A, Ramakrishna H. Analysis of Conduction Abnormalities and Permanent Pacemaker Implantation After Transcatheter Aortic Valve Replacement. Journal of Cardiothoracic and Vascular Anesthesia. 2020 Apr 1;34(4):1082-93.

[26] Fujita B, Schmidt T, Bleiziffer S, Bauer T, Beckmann A, Bekeredjian R, Möllmann H, Walther T, Landwehr S, Hamm C, Beyersdorf F. Impact of new pacemaker implantation following surgical and transcatheter aortic valve replacement on 1-year outcome. European Journal of Cardio-Thoracic Surgery. 2020 Jan 1;57(1):151-9.

[27] Mazzella AJ, Hendrickson MJ, Arora S, Sanders M, Li Q, Vavalle JP, Gehi AK. Shifting Trends in Timing of Pacemaker Implantation After Transcatheter Aortic Valve Replacement. Cardiovascular Interventions. 2020 Nov 9.

[28] Pollari F, Dell'Aquila AM, Söhn C, Marianowicz J, Wiehofsky P, Schwab J, Pauschinger M, Hitzl W, Fischlein T, Pfeiffer S. Risk factors for paravalvular leak after transcatheter aortic valve replacement. The Journal of thoracic and cardiovascular surgery. 2019 Apr 1;157(4):1406-15.

[29] Leon MB, Smith CR, Mack MJ, Makkar RR, Svensson LG, Kodali SK, Thourani VH, Tuzcu EM, Miller DC, Herrmann HC, Doshi D. Transcatheter or surgical aortic-valve replacement in intermediate-risk patients. New England Journal of Medicine. 2016 Apr 28;374(17):1609-20.

[30] Armoiry X, Obadia JF, Iung B, Polazzi S, Duclos A. Clinical outcomes and direct costs after transcatheter aortic valve implantation in French centres: a longitudinal study of 1332 patients using a national database. Interactive cardiovascular and thoracic surgery. 2016 Dec 1;23(6):883-8.

[31] Baron SJ, Wang K, House JA, Magnuson EA, Reynolds MR, Makkar R, Herrmann HC, Kodali S, Thourani VH, Kapadia S, Svensson L. Cost-effectiveness of transcatheter versus surgical aortic valve replacement in patients with severe aortic stenosis at intermediate risk: results from the PARTNER 2 trial. Circulation. 2019 Feb 12;139(7):877-88.

[32] El-Haddad H, Resar J. Stenting the Snorkel: PCI of a Restenosed Left Main Stent Placed for Coronary Obstruction after Valve in Valve TAVR. Journal of Structural Heart Disease. 2019 Apr;5(2):48-51.

[33] Voudris KV, Petropulos P, Karyofillis P, Charitakis K. Timing and Outcomes of PCI in the TAVR Era. Current treatment options in cardiovascular medicine. 2018 Mar 1;20(3):22.

[34] Faroux L, Campelo-Parada F, Munoz-Garcia E, Nombela-Franco L, Fischer Q, Donaint P, Serra V, Veiga G, Gutiérrez E, Vilalta V, Alperi A. Procedural Characteristics and Late Outcomes of Percutaneous Coronary Intervention in the Workup Pre-TAVR. JACC: Cardiovascular Interventions. 2020 Oct 14.

[35] Tarus A, Tinica G, Bacusca A, Artene B, Popa IV, Burlacu A. Coronary revascularization during treatment of severe aortic stenosis: A meta-analysis of the complete percutaneous approach (PCI plus TAVR) versus the complete surgical approach (CABG plus SAVR). Journal of Cardiac Surgery. 2020 Aug;35(8):2009-16.

[36] Goldstone AB, Chiu P, Baiocchi M, Lingala B, Patrick WL, Fischbein MP, Woo YJ. Mechanical or biologic prostheses for aortic-valve and mitral-valve replacement. New England Journal of Medicine. 2017 Nov 9;377(19):1847-57.

[37] Nishimura RA, Otto CM, Bonow RO, Carabello BA, Erwin JP, Fleisher LA, Jneid H, Mack MJ, McLeod CJ, O'Gara PT, Rigolin VH. 2017 AHA/ACC focused update of the 2014 AHA/ACC guideline for the management of patients with valvular heart disease: a report of the American College of Cardiology/American Heart Association Task Force on Clinical Practice Guidelines. Journal of the American College of Cardiology. 2017 Jul 3;70(2):252-89.

[38] James TM, Stamou SC, Rothenberg M, Nores MA. Transcatheter aortic valve in valve implantation with bioprosthetic valve fracture. Catheterization and Cardiovascular Interventions. 2019 May 1;93(6):1170-2.

[39] Coylewright M, Forrest JK, McCabe JM, Nazif TM. TAVR in low-risk patients: FDA approval, the new NCD, and shared decision-making. Journal of the American College of Cardiology. 2020 Mar 17;75(10):1208-11.

Chapter 2

Aortic Valve Disease: State of the Art

Adam El Gamel

Abstract

Aortic valve replacement is the most commonly performed valve operation. It has been shown to be an effective therapy in all age groups, including the very elderly (age > 90 years). The most common etiologies for aortic stenosis are calcific degeneration, rheumatic disease, and congenital bicuspid valves. The most common causes of pure aortic regurgitation include annuloaortic ectasia and associated dilation of the aortic root, endocarditis, aortic dissection, and rheumatic disease. The indications for surgery depend on the pathophysiology and symptoms. The choice of the prosthesis can be difficult and depends on multiple clinical and lifestyle considerations. Early and late outcomes are generally quite good, even in high-risk patients.

Keywords: aortic valve, aortic stenosis, aortic incompetence, valve replacement, TAVI, aortic valve repair

1. Introduction

Valve disease still a significant health problem in the developed countries, In United states nearly 2.5% of the population has moderate or severe valve disease, with increased the prevalence for people older than 64 years and is 13% in those older than 75 years [1].

The commonest valve diseases in the elderly are calcific aortic valve disease and aortic dilation causing aortic regurgitation [2].

While rheumatic heart disease is the most prevalent pathology of valve disease globally, especially in the adolescent and young adults with a projected prevalence of 16–20 million, rheumatic fever is the most frequent trigger of valve disease in the young, particularly in Africa, India, the Middle East, South America, and parts of Australia and New Zealand, China, and Russia [3]. In western countries, the incidence of rheumatic disease declined in the latter half of the twentieth century, with the occurrence of transitory local episodes. In Africa, endomyocardial fibrosis is a common, poorly investigated pathology that leads to valve disease in all ages [4]. On the other hand, in the developed countries valve diseases of elderly predominate, particularly calcific aortic stenosis and functional mitral regurgitation, with a prevalence of 13% in those older than 75 years reported in North America [5–7].

Other pathological conditions like infective endocarditis and drug-induced valve disease (5-HT2B receptor agonists) are on the rise [8–10].

IntechOpen

Structural biological valves deterioration would be the future burden on health resources world-wide; this is due to its current popularity as a therapeutic option even in young patients, mainly to avoid the complications of anticoagulation [11, 12].

Lack of equitable access to health care takes place in all countries, as a consequence of many complex economic and social forces. Because of the escalating technological cost of health care around the world, the situation is the same, even those industrially developed countries.

The salient global errand is the prevention of rheumatic heart disease, which would necessitate cooperation among social, political, and medical programs that lead to creating enhancements in living conditions by better housing, nutrition and improved access to health care [13–16]. Penicillin for streptococcal throat infections and secondary prophylaxis would continue to be a cornerstone in the global fight against rheumatic heart disease [17–19]. It is also reported that there was a natural reduction in the virulence of streptococcal serotypes, but it happened after the incidence of rheumatic fever had declined.

Most of the serum biomarkers that have been shown related to VHD are detecting secondary effects on the ventricular myocardium. Biomarkers associated with myocardial stress include the natriuretic peptides and GDF-15. Troponin is linked to myocardial necrosis, and the micro RNAs, ST2, and galectin-3 are associated with myocardial hypertrophy and fibrosis. Of these, the natriuretic peptides are the most widely studied, but they are not specific to VHD, and there is considerable overlap in serum levels between different clinical groups [20–22].

2. Practical anatomy and physiology of the aortic valve

The aortic valve is the last gate the blood pumped from the heart to the rest of the organs. It is at the junction between the aorta and the outflow tract of the left ventricle. Its function is to maintain unidirectional blood flow during the diastole while allowing the blood forward flow with minimal resistance during systole. The aortic valve has typically three semilunar cusps (tricuspid) named by their relationship to the coronary Ostia: the left coronary and right coronary, and the third is the noncoronary cusp. Cusps are attached to the aortic annulus at the bottom of slight dilations of the aorta associated with each cusp (sinuses of Valsalva end at the sinotubular junction). The sinotubular junction is the narrowest part of the aortic

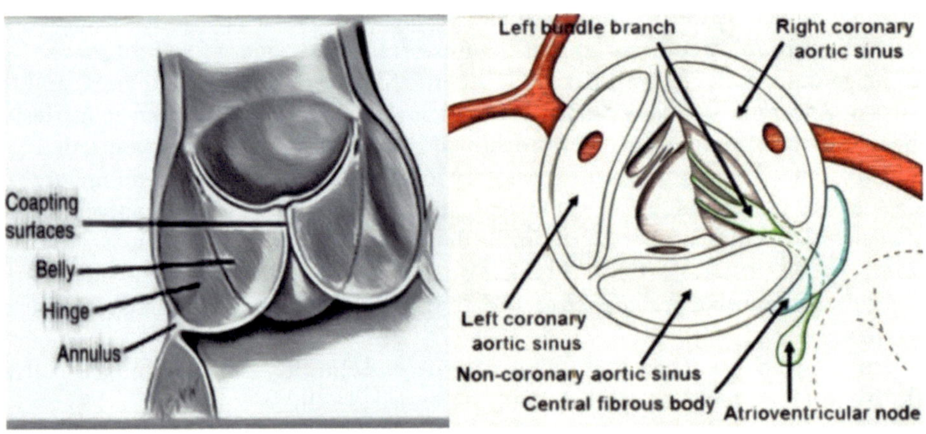

Figure 1.
Aortic valve anatomy.

root (**Figure 1**). The fibrous skeleton supports the aortic valve and is continuous with the anterior leaflet of the mitral valve [23, 24].

3. Managing a patient with suspected valvular heart disease

3.1 General principles

Detection of valvular heart disorder can be difficult. The state of the patient may range in gravity from asymptomatic to cardiogenic shock. Endocarditis may mimic systemic illness, vascular or neurologic condition, while acute aortic incompetence may be presented as a primary respiratory disorder (acute asthmatic episode). Making a timely, accurate diagnosis, while averting excessive laboratory studies, may try the acumen of a seasoned clinician.

Commonly, observing a murmur in a well individual or a patient with symptom referable to the cardiovascular system, arouse the suspicion of valvular abnormality. It is essential to reassure the patients; murmur is not synonymous with heart disease. It does represent turbulent blood flow which may result from several possible conditions. These include: (i) increased flow secondary to anaemia, pregnancy, or a hyperadrenergic state; accelerated flow through a restricted orifice (ii) regurgitant flow through a leaking valve; or (iii) abnormal shunting between two chambers. In an unselected population, most systolic murmurs are physiologic, caused by conditions of increased blood flow [25, 26]. The echocardiogram is the best way to evaluate the patients and reassure them [27, 28].

The practical approach to these patients relies upon an open-minded history and thorough physical examination.

3.2 History

As in nearly all of medicine, most cues to a diagnosis are from history.

The clinician assessment should not be compromised, trying to spare minutes at this stage drain hours in the wasted investigation later.

The patient may provide a history of rheumatic fever, pervious episode of infective endocarditis, intravenous drug use, use of anorectic medications, carcinoid tumours, indwelling vascular devices, dental, genitourinary or gastrointestinal procedures; Marfan's syndrome, syphilis; congenital bicuspid aortic valve; treated or untreated coronary artery disease, radiation therapy.

Finally, a history of past surgery increases the risk of future valve problems by way of prosthetic valve endocarditis or structural failure.

Family genetics undoubtedly plays a role in so doing; the clinician may identify a family with a previously unrecognised genetic mutation and allowed early diagnosis of relatives. The social history may provide valuable information. For example, a childhood spent in a no industrialised region of the world dramatically increases the risk of rheumatic valve disease. History of unprotected sex or intravenous drug abuse raises the TE.

Course for valvular heart disease varies widely, ranging from minutes to decades dependent on primary pathology and age and risk factors related to patients as well as the geographical location in the world.

3.2.1 Dyspnea

Unfortunately, it is also very nonspecific, occurring in nearly any disturbance of cardiopulmonary function. Orthopnoea and paroxysmal nocturnal dyspnea are somewhat more specific for left ventricular failure.

3.2.2 Palpitations

The sensation of a rapid or unusually vigorous heartbeat may signal the development of atrial fibrillation.

3.2.3 Angina

Maybe the initial manifestation of valvular heart disease.

3.2.4 Weight gain, oedema, and abdominal discomfort

In hospitalised patients, excess extra cellular fluid is first presented as pitting oedema overlying the sacrum predominantly; the elevated systemic venous pressure is the cause of all the above.

3.3 Physical exam

3.3.1 General appearance

The toxic appearance of acute infection, wasting of cardiac cachexia, the distressed facial expression, wet cough, accessory muscle use, and diaphoresis of pulmonary oedema, and the cool skin characteristic of poor perfusion.

3.3.2 Vital signs

3.3.2.1 Tachycardia

Skin and mucosa cyanosis of the lips cold sweat (Osler nodes). (Janeway lesions), painless red macule lesions of the palms and soles (Janeway lesions), conjunctive petechial, and subungual hematomas (splinter haemorrhages).

Central venous pulsations jugular venous pulsation and mean central venous pressure (CVP) are often abnormal in valvular heart disease. In most cases, right heart failure is secondary left-sided valve disease-causing left heart failure. Less direct clues to the level of right atrial pressure; include the presence of pedal oedema, sacral oedema, anasarca, tender hepatomegaly, ecchymosis (hepatic synthetic dysfunction), hepatojugular pulsation and ascites.

3.3.3 Pulse volume, contour

3.3.3.1 Auscultatory findings

However, auscultation technical skill like any other and improves with repetition [29]. Therefore, students' physicians-in-training reading this text should lose heart, but rather, should apply themselves diligently to acquire these valuable bedside skills. Listening to patients before and after echocardiographic findings are known is particularly helpful.

3.4 Electrocardiography

In majority of patients with aortic valve disease with have abnormal ECG which commonly non-specific such as left ventricle hypertrophy, with or without repolarization abnormalities is seen on electrocardiography (ECG). Left atrial enlargement, left axis deviation and conduction disorders are also common. Atrial fibrillation can be seen at late state and in older patients or those with hypertension.

3.5 Radiography

Pulmonary vascular congestion. Enlargement, valvular calcification, and type position of prosthetic valve may all be ascertained plain radiographs. Comparing changes over time particularly helpful; hence obtaining previous studies is very valuable (**Figure 2**).

3.6 Echocardiography

Echocardiography is the most valuable tool in valvular heart disease due to its portability, ease of use. Low cost, steadily improving resolution, and its ability to assess hemodynamics, additional ultrasound-based modalities can provide information about cardiac anatomy, function, and hemodynamics. These modalities include two dimensional (2D) or B-mode in which sound waves are in a fan-like distribution, yielding a real wedge-shaped tomographic image of the heart. There are three subtypes of Doppler ultrasound. Continuous-wave Doppler, all velocities along a continuous line through the heart are displayed as a spectrum over time. In pulse wave Doppler, the sample volume is placed on a 2D image, and the spectral splay of velocities represents the blood flow velocities in this region only.

Tissue Doppler is yet another form of Doppler echocardiography which measures the velocity of anatomic structures rather than red blood cells; it currently has very limited application in valvular heart disease [30, 31].

Hemodynamic assessment. Firstly, the pressure gradient a valve or between two chambers can be estimated by taking advantage of the relationship between pressure (P), and velocity (v) as described in is the conservation of flow and different diameter, the flow of fluid through one section match flow through the other end. Since flow equals the product of orifice area and flow velocity, this principle can be stated as Area 1 × Velocity 1 = Area 2 × Velocity 2. This is used explicitly in the determination of aortic valve area (**Figure 3**) [30].

Another hemodynamic measure important valvular heart disease are the rate of pressure equilibration between two chambers (e.g. pressure half-time, deceleration).

Cardiac catheterisation and direct measure of intracardiac pressures, ventriculography, aortography, and assessment of coronary vessels before valve surgery all continue to be an essential tool in the evaluation of valvular heart disease.

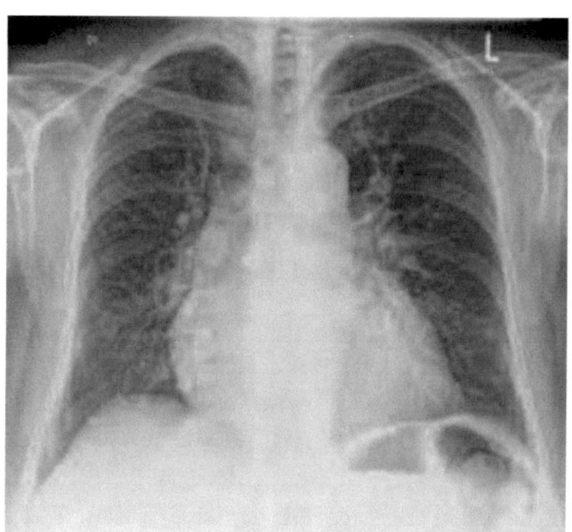

Figure 2.
Cardiomegaly and pulmonary congestion.

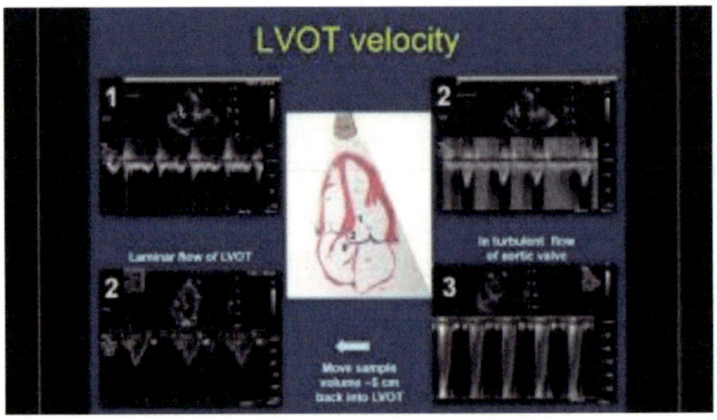

Figure 3.
Echocardiogram assessment of aortic valve.

Occasionally, balloon valvotomy serves an important therapeutic and diagnostic role in mitral, and occasionally, aortic stenosis.

Positron emission tomography (PET) is an emerging imaging technique which allows improved resolution more flexibility than SPECT, including the possibility of imaging metabolic substrates and neural transmitters. In light of its expense and dependency mostly cyclotron-produced isotopes, its role in valvular heart disease remains to be determined.

3.7 Aortic stenosis

Aortic stenosis (AS) may be to congenital or acquired, and the congenital form could be above (supra), below (subvalvular) or at the valve level. A supravalvular is a rare form of long and tubular narrowing is associated with, (William's Syndrome) hypercalcemia, mental retardation, and peripheral pulmonic stenosis. Subvalvular stenosis may be caused by the septum extending into the outflow tract, a cylindrical constriction of the outflow tract or, in hypertrophic cardiomyopathy the obstruction caused by the anterior movement of the mitral valve leaflets. In some patients, this is present only at diminished ventricular (LV) volumes recreated in the echocardiography laboratory by Valsalva cause aortic regurgitation [32].

3.8 Epidemiology and aetiology

Isolated aortic stenosis (AS) is more frequent in men and is found in 2% of people 65 years of age and older. The most frequent causes of AS include age-related calcific degeneration, bicuspid aortic valve, and rheumatic aortic valve. The distribution of these causes diverges across age groups and geographic regions. Age-related degeneration is the commonest cause of AS in elderly patients. In comparison, bicuspid aortic valve calcification accounts for most surgical cases in younger patients (>65) [33].

3.9 Pathophysiology

There is 0 gradient exists across the standard aortic valve during the cardiac cycle. The cross-sectional area of a normal aortic valve is >2 cm^2. While reductions in the valve area to 1.5–2.0 leads to minimal pressure gradient, further narrowing produces dramatic increases in the mean pressure gradient [34]. In AS, progressive obstruction of outflow tract increases afterload ventricular, and wall stress of the left ventricle leads to high left ventricular systolic and diastolic pressures, decreased aortic pressure, and prolonged left ventricular ejection time.

Obstruction to flow usually develops slowly allowing the LV to adapt by concentric thickening hypertrophy serves to reduce wall tension (the law of Laplace describes wall tension is proportional to pressure and radius and adversely proportional to thickness). As long as the process of muscular wall thickening keeps pace with narrowing of the aortic orifice, the 'wall tension' is maintained. Gradually, this results in compensatory concentric left ventricular hypertrophy (LVH) to maintain ejection fraction [35].

The stability comes at a price, now the hypertrophied walls are less compliant and LV less able to fill rapidly. Satisfactory end-diastolic volume becomes heavily reliant upon atrial contraction. Atrial fibrillation often precipitates dramatic acute congestive heart failure in patients with severe AS. The concentric hypertrophy increases myocardial oxygen requirement coupled with reduced coronary flow due to deviated diastole and low diastolic pressures, which aggravates subendocardial ischemia in the presence of normal coronary artery ventricular arrhythmias are common as well. The compensatory mechanism may become insufficient in patients with chronic severe AS, resulting in thinning and dilation of the left ventricle, leading to a decrease in ejection fraction and congestive heart failure [36].

Exertional syncope may develop resulting from peripheral vasodilation induced by exercise with the background of a fixed cardiac output. Blood pressure drop may reduce cerebral perfusion, below the minimum required for consciousness [37].

A negative balance between oxygen supply and demand is the norm in AS. LVH increased afterload, and the long systole increases myocardial oxygen demand. The high filling pressure and longer systolic time decrease myocardial oxygen supply by reducing myocardial perfusion time. Myocardial ischemia in patients with AS is due to the alteration in myocardial oxygen supply and demand even in the absence of coronary artery disease.

3.10 Clinical features

3.10.1 Clinical presentation

3.10.1.1 Symptoms

Patients with, mild or moderate AS are usually asymptomatic unless they have the coexisting cardiopulmonary disease or infective endocarditis. Patients often remain asymptomatic until the ventricle begins to fail. At this initially, they usually develop fatigue followed by cardinal symptoms of angina, syncope, and dyspnea expected survival following the onset of these symptoms is 2, 3, and 5 years, respectively [38].

In rare instances, sudden tragic death is the first manifestation of the disease. Patients may be sedentary; it unclear whether they are inactive by choice or have gradually restricted their activity to avoid symptoms. A treadmill stress test under close medical supervision may help in their assessment.

3.10.1.2 Physical findings

The classic finding in the assessment of peripheral pulses is a delayed and slowly rising wave contour pulsus parvus et tardus. However, it may be absent patients with associated aortic regurgitation or in patients with associated aortic regurgitation or calcified, inelastic arteries.

Precordial palpation may reveal a sustained and laterally displaced cardiac impulse. Because the hypertrophied LV is noncompliant, the critical contribution to filling provided by atrial contraction severe thrill is often palpable at the base of the heart.

3.10.2 Ejection systolic crescendo murmur at the second aortic area

3.10.2.1 Electrocardiogram

Standard features on the electrocardiogram include ventricular hypertrophy (LVH) with a strain and a biphasic p wave in V1 corresponding to atrial (LA) hypertrophy. Atrioventricular and intra ventricular conduction abnormalities maybe when calcification extends from the valve into the induction system.

3.10.2.2 Radiography

The chest X-ray rounding of the left heart border and apex, post stenotic dilation of the aorta calcification of the aortic valve, and pulmonary congestion may be apparent. Note, these findings are neither highly sensitive nor specific.

3.10.2.3 Echocardiography

Echocardiography serves as the principal modality for and quantitating AS. 2D imaging provides information on chamber size, degree of hypertrophy, LV systolic function, valve mobility, and calcification. Doppler measurement of transvalvular blood flow velocity can be used to ermine peak and mean pressure gradients using the.

The symptomatic triad of AS is angina, exertional syncope, and symptoms of congestive heart failure, such as shortness of breath. The mechanisms for angina and congestive heart failure are explained in the previous section. The mechanism for syncope is likely related to the blunting of exercise-induced augmentation in stroke volume as a result of outflow obstruction coupled with exercise-induced peripheral vasodilation. These changes cause a drop in systemic blood pressure leading to cerebral hypoperfusion and syncope.

The classic physical finding is a systolic ejection murmur heard loudest at the second right intercostal space, which commonly radiates to the carotid arteries. And maybe associated with severe cases of AS palpable thrill may be present. Palpation of the pulse may reveal a weak and delayed pulse known as *pulsus parvus et tardus*.

3.11 Diagnosis and grading

The most common method for the diagnosis and grading of AS is two-dimensional transthoracic echocardiography Doppler velocity measurement (**Table 1**). In most patients, this modality can reliably establish aortic jet velocity, aortic valve peak and mean gradients, and aortic valve area [39].

3.12 Natural history

Without valve replacement symptomatic AS has a bleak outcome. Numerous studies consistently reported survivals of 3 years for angina and syncope and 1.5–2 years for dyspnea and heart failure. These findings have determined the recommendations for timely surgical intervention in patients with symptomatic AS. Thirty percent of truly asymptomatic severe AS patients will become symptomatic in 2 years with mortality risks of less than 1–5% each year to 5% each year. Progression rate correlates with AS severity, which seems to progress faster with higher mean gradient. Moderate AS progress, with aortic valve area, decreases on average by 0.1 cm^2 per cent annually the pressure gradient across the valve rises on average by 7 mm Hg per year, and the jet velocity increases by 0.3 m/s per year [40, 41].

Parameter	Mild	Moderate	Severe
Aortic valve area (cm^2)	1.6–2.5	1.1–1.5	≤1.0
Mean pressure gradient (mm Hg)	<20	20–39	≥40
Aortic jet velocity (m/s)	2.0–2.9	3.0–3.9	≥4.0

Table 1.
The severity of aortic stenosis according to echocardiographic criteria.

The definitions of the conditions "low-gradient AS" and "high-gradient AS" are the most relevant new changes in the recommendations for the management of aortic valve stenosis (AS). Precise thresholds of biomarkers and pulmonary hypertension are considered, and the emphasis is focused on computed tomography, particularly for assessing the degree of calcification of the aortic valve and for planning therapy [42].

3.13 Aortic regurgitation

3.13.1 Epidemiology and aetiology

The reasons of aortic regurgitation (AR) are many and can be credited to a disruption of any components of the functional unit of the aortic root valve composite (e.g., cusps, sinuses of Valsalva, sinotubular junction, annulus). In general, the causes can be divided into those that involve the valve cusps (e.g., calcific degeneration, congenitally bicuspid valve, infective endocarditis, rheumatic disease, myxomatous degeneration) and those that encompass the aortic root (e.g., aortic dissection, aortitis of various etiologies such as syphilis, connective tissue disorders such as Marfan syndrome) [43].

3.13.2 Pathophysiology

The pathophysiology of AR is determined by the speed of onset and duration of the disease process. In acute AR, typically caused by aortic dissection, infective endocarditis, trauma, or valve prosthesis failure, there is an abrupt escalation in left ventricular end-diastolic volume because of the regurgitation. Since the left ventricle has restricted compliance and does not have enough time to gradually adapt to the extra volume, the left ventricular end-diastolic pressure (LVEDP) rises rapidly [44, 45].

In chronic AR, there is a gradual and stealthy evolution of left ventricular (LV) dilation and eccentric hypertrophy because of an increase in left ventricular end-diastolic volume, LVEDP, and wall stress. Dilation of the LV maintains normal systolic function and forward flow but requiring extra work to achieve normality. Sooner or later, the hypertrophic response is exhausted, and LVEF deteriorates as afterload increases, resulting in heart failure and its related clinical presentation [44].

3.13.3 Clinical features

Patients with acute AR present with unexpected or precipitously cardiovascular collapse, which is a life-threatening emergency. They often demonstrate ischemic symptoms because of the diminished coronary blood flow and heightened myocardial oxygen demand. In comparison, patients with chronic AR are often asymptomatic for an extended time because of the compensator remodelling of their LV mentioned earlier. Once the compensatory response is depleted, the patients experience heart failure symptoms such as exertional dyspnea, orthopnea, and paroxysmal nocturnal dyspnea. Patients may also suffer palpitations and angina [46].

The classic murmur of AR is an early diastolic, blowing, a decrescendo murmur heard best at the level of the diaphragm at the left sternal border while the patient is sitting, leaning forward, and in deep exhalation.

Classic signs of widened pulse pressure may also be found, including Corrigan or water-hammer pulse, De Musset sign (bobbing of the head with heartbeats), Quincke pulse (pulsations of the lip and fingers), Traube sign (pistol shot sounds over the femoral artery), and Müller sign (pulsations of the uvula).

3.13.4 Diagnostic criteria

Transthoracic echocardiography with Doppler colour-flow is the most useful tool for the diagnosis of AR. The jet width and vena contracta width on Doppler colour-flow are used to qualitatively assess the severity of AR, whereas the regurgitant volume, regurgitant fraction, and regurgitant orifice area are used for the quantitative assessment.

3.13.5 Management of aortic valve disease

3.13.5.1 Medical management

Many adverse outcomes in adults with valvular heart disease are due to sequelae of the disease process, including atrial fibrillation, embolic events, left ventricular (LV) dysfunction, pulmonary hypertension, and endocarditis. Patients with valvular heart disease are best cared for in the context of a multidisciplinary heart valve clinic [47].

Medical therapy in adults with valvular heart disease focuses on prevention and treatment of complications because there are no specific therapies to prevent progression of the valve disease itself apart from primary and secondary prophylaxis of rheumatic fever. Rheumatic fever is a multiorgan inflammatory disease that occurs 10 days to 3 weeks after group A streptococcal pharyngitis. The clinical diagnosis is based on the conjunction of an antecedent streptococcal throat infection and classic manifestations of the disease, including carditis, polyarthritis, chorea, erythema marginatum, and subcutaneous nodules [48]. Reducing the frequency of streptococcal pharyngitis with benzylpenicillin monthly intramuscular injection helps to reduce the progression of Rheumatic heart disease. The risk of recurrent disease is related to the number of previous episodes, time interval since the last episode, the risk of exposure to streptococcal infections (contact with children or crowded situations), and patient age. A longer duration of secondary prevention is recommended in patients with evidence of carditis or persistent valvular disease than in those with no evidence of valvular damage [49].

Endocarditis prophylaxis guidelines recommend antibiotics therapy before dental procedures, or other procedures associated with bacteraemia, in adults with prosthetic valves but not in patients with native valve disease unless the patient had an episode of endocarditis, dental hygiene and gum health are the primary preventive measure to reduce endocarditis [50].

Prevention of embolic events in patients with valvular heart disease, particularly those with prosthetic valves, MS, or AF, is a key component of optimal medical therapy.

Therapy for the prevention of embolic events in patients with valvular heart disease typically includes antiplatelet agents or long-term warfarin anticoagulation [51, 52]. There is data on the use of newer anticoagulants, such as direct thrombin inhibitors and anti-Xa agents, for prevention of embolic events in patients with valve disease [53]. At the initiation of therapy, a target INR and acceptable range are defined by the referring physician for each patient on the basis of published guidelines and clinical factors unique to that patient, In addition, patient education about anticoagulation, possible dietary and drug interactions, recognition of complications of therapy, and the need for careful monitoring of the INR is provided verbally and through the use of a variety of media (such as pamphlets, recorded presentations, and computer-based material).

Periodic evaluation of disease severity by echocardiography and clinical evaluation of the LV response to chronic volume and/or pressure overload allows optimal timing of surgical and percutaneous interventions. General health maintenance is important, including evaluation and treatment of coronary disease risk factors, regular exercise, standard immunisations. Both pneumococcal and annual influenza vaccinations are recommended for all adults older than 65 years and are especially important in patients with valvular disease, in whom the increased hemodynamic demands of acute infection may lead to cardiac decompensation. In younger patients with valve disease, routine immunisation is only indicated in conditions associated with immunocompromise are also present and optimal dental care. Management of concurrent cardiovascular disease follows standard approaches with modification, as needed, based on the potential confounding effects of valve haemodynamics. Evaluation of coronary anatomy usually is needed before valve surgery because of the high prevalence of coronary disease and improved surgical outcomes with concurrent coronary revascularisation.

Periodic noninvasive monitoring is essential for the optimal timing of interventions in patients with valve dysfunction. Disease progression may be evident as changes in valve anatomy or motion; an increase in the severity of valve stenosis or regurgitation; LV dilation, hypertrophy, or dysfunction in response to pressure and/or volume overload; or secondary effects of the valvular lesion, such as pulmonary hypertension or AF.

Although the goal in the management of patients with valvular disease is to avoid symptoms and the need for medical therapy by optimising the timing of surgical intervention, some patients have persistent symptoms after surgery, have symptoms only in response to superimposed hemodynamic stress (such as pregnancy), or are not candidates for surgical intervention. In these situations, medical therapy is based primarily on adjustment of loading conditions and control of heart rate and rhythm.

Most adverse outcomes of noncardiac surgery in adults with valve disease are due to failure to recognise the presence of valve disease preoperatively. When valve disease is suspected from history or physical examination findings, echocardiography is appropriate to identify and define the severity of any valve lesions. In patients with valvular disease undergoing noncardiac surgery, management focuses on an accurate assessment of disease severity and symptom status, with appropriate hemodynamic monitoring and optimisation of loading conditions in the perioperative period [54].

3.13.5.2 Patient education

Patient education is the key to compliance with periodic noninvasive monitoring, prevention of complications, and the early recognition of symptoms in patients with valvular heart disease. Each patient should understand the expected long-term prognosis, potential complications, typical symptoms, the rationale for sequential monitoring, and the indications for surgical intervention. Appropriate education avoids needless concern and prompts early reporting of symptoms, allowing optimal timing of surgical intervention. Increasingly, patients are actively involved in decisions about the timing of surgery and choice of intervention.

Patients also should be knowledgeable about the risk of infective endocarditis and the importance of maintaining optimal oral hygiene, including regular dental care.

Patients undergoing long-term anticoagulation need both education and a reliable and available source for consultation regarding warfarin dose, interactions with other medications, and prompt evaluation of any complications.

3.13.5.3 Aortic valve replacement

The decision for intervention for a faulty aortic valve needs to incorporate the natural history of the medically managed disease, the risks associated with the intervention, and longer-term problems that might build up as a result of prosthetic valve implantation.

Currently, the heart team plays a decisive role in decision making. In addition, it is prudent to cultivate and set up heart valve centres with specialist services in order to generate an ideal environment for the treatment of patients with valvular heart disease.

3.13.5.4 Management of Aortic valve stenosis

Criteria for decision-making are clear for surgical valve and transcatheter aortic valve implantation (TAVI) from the current European guidelines. Recently TAVI is also recommended for patients with intermediate surgical risk. Currently, publish literature also supports TAVI implantation in low risk patients as non-inferior to surgical therapy [55, 56].

For symptomatic, AS recommendations are made with regard to the choice of procedure. For high risk (STS score or EuroSCORE II <4% or a log EuroSCORE <10%) TAVI is the default choice. Surgical replacement is indicated for patients with a low perioperative risk (STS score > 4%). Patients with an intermediate surgical risk, the heart team, should consider other criteria for decision making such as anatomical and functional parameters [57, 58], and frailty to reach the best option for the patients considering the current knowledge.

Current data from two large prospective randomised studies, have confirmed that TAVI was noninferior to surgical treatment with regard to mortality, stroke and additional endpoints in both in patients with a low perioperative risk (the mean STS score in both trials was 1.9%), expansion of the indication for TAVI which would also include younger patients, can be expected [59].

3.13.6 Choice of a valve in surgically treated patients

3.13.6.1 Choice of prosthesis

Choice of prosthesis is a complex decision in a patient undergoing AVR with profound long-term consequences for the patient. Currently available prostheses are different with regard to key features, such as the requirement of anticoagulation, incidence of thromboembolism, durability, ease of implantation, haemodynamic performance, and susbtibilty for infection. Currently age-based guidelines do exist, but the final choice must be tailored to the individual patient including consideration of general lifestyle and physical activity, surgeon expertise, diseases, especially those affecting life expectancy, and, ultimately, overall patient preference.

The patient age is a primary factor in prosthesis selection is. Elderly patients have lower life expectancy and physical activity than Younger patients. Which place a greater demand on the prosthesis with regard to durability and hemodynamic performance. Age has long been recognised as a major determinant of bioprosthesis durability. Traditionally target age between 65 and 70 years has been the indications for bioprosthesis and like hood of a second operation for structural valve dysfunction in a life time 65-year-old person is less than 10%. As a result, it is not common to choose a mechanical valve in an old patient. Even if the patient is already treated with warfarin for another condition, for example AF, which should not necessarily favour the choice of a mechanical valve because it converts a relative indication for low-level anticoagulation to an absolute indication for higher levels. It also removes the option to stop warfarin in a case of a significant bleeding event. Moreover even if the patient had previously received mechanical valve, the choice does not mandate a second mechanical valve, because risk of complications thromboembolic and bleeding is higher with two mechanical valves than it is with one.

It is more complex and controversial to choose of prosthesis in patients younger than 65 years. Although traditionally, these patients would receive a mechanical valve; the current, improved durability in bioprosthesis and lower operative risk of a redo operation for a failed prosthesis have increased the number of patients younger than 65 years who receive bioprosthesis, including patients in their 50s and even younger.

A particular dilemma women of child-bearing age often it is safer avoid warfarin so they choose a bioprosthesis, with the knowledge that they will face at least one reoperation in their lifetime.

Stentless valves may provide a larger effective orifice area such as the Toronto SPV, Freestyle, and Prima Plus valves although the hemodynamic profiles of stentless valves are superior to those of stented valves, especially at the smaller sizes [42] durability and survival benefits still is unproven [47, 48]. Some reports suggest fewer thromboembolic complications [49]. Currently no specifics indication form stentless valve. Maybe these hemodynamic benefits justify implanting stentless valves in younger active patients.

The use of homografts has declined in recent years as a primary aortic valve substitute because without a durability advantage, it is cumbersome to recommend their routine while they have limited availability and the cumbersome storage requirements. However, their ability to resist infection renders them an excellent solution for patients with endocarditis.

The Ross procedure involves replacing the aortic valve with the patient's own pulmonic valve, which have to be is replaced with a homograft or a stentless xenograft. The benefits are near-normal haemodynamic and excellent durability; the disadvantages are the technical complexity and need for reoperation for the homograft or Late AR. The procedure peaked in popularity in the mid to late 1990s, but procedure volume has declined since then. On the basis of the data from the Ross Procedure International Registry, several centres continue to report excellent results [50, 51] although it is now primarily a procedure for paediatric patients, in whom the potential for growth is important, and for young adults in their 20s and 30s when no other good alternatives exist.

3.13.7 Special situations

3.13.7.1 Low-flow, low-gradient aortic valve

The precise assessment within the heart team of the pathology and anatomy, as well as the evaluation of the patient, are emphasised in the new graduated recommendations regarding low-flow, low-gradient aortic valve stenosis in symptomatic patients [60].

It is also highly recommended to take into account the morphology of the device landing zone and the resulting individual risks for TAVI procedures.

For asymptomatic patients with an indication for aortic valve replacement, surgical replacement is still the gold standard, because no data are available for this patient cohort concerning TAVI treatment.

3.13.7.2 Management of aortic regurgitation

Surgical aortic valve replacement remains the standard gold treatment of aortic valve regurgitation (AR). Transcatheter aortic valve implantation (TAVI) plays only a minor role. Currently, the JenaValve (JenaValve Technology GmbH, Munich, Germany) is the only prosthesis available for pure AR as an investigational device [61]. All other prostheses are used off label [61]. Concerning the choice of the type of prosthesis, criteria used in aortic stenosis are not merely interchangeable. The percentage of oversizing has to be calculated in a different way because of the absence annular calcification. Although outcomes have improved with newer-generation TAVI devices outcomes are still inferior to surgery. In a few circumstances, TAVI might be an option for patients with severe AR and high surgical risk.

The class I recommendations for aortic valve intervention, in patients with AR according to the 2014 American College of Cardiology and the American Heart Association are the following: symptomatic patients with chronic severe AR, asymptomatic patients with chronic severe AR and LV dysfunction (ejection fraction < 50%) at rest, and patients with chronic severe AR who are undergoing concomitant coronary artery bypass grafting, aortic surgery, or other heart valve surgery.

The class IIa recommendation is for patients with asymptomatic AR and normal LV systolic function (ejection fraction > 50%) but with severe LV dilation (end-systolic diameter > 50 mm). The class IIb recommendation is for patients with moderate AR who are undergoing coronary artery bypass grafting, aortic surgery, or other heart valve surgery. Aortic valve intervention may also be reasonable in asymptomatic patients with chronic severe AR, normal LV systolic function, and severe LV dilation (end-diastolic diameter > 65 mm) if the operative risk is low. Other considerations can include evidence of progressive LV dilation, declining exercise tolerance, or abnormal hemodynamic response to exercise [62, 63].

However, aortic valve repair carries a similar, if not lower, risk of perioperative complication with a low risk of valve-related events over time. Similar to mitral valve repair for mitral regurgitation, [six] there is some suggestion that aortic valve intervention should be considered earlier in patients in whom aortic valve repair is likely [64].

Another broad category of patients who undergo aortic valve preservation and repair are those with primary aortic pathology involving the aortic root or the ascending aorta and varying degrees of associated aortic valvular disease. In these patients, the primary indication for intervention is driven by aortic size, discussed in the American, European, and Canadian Guidelines.

From a technical perspective, all patients with primary aortic insufficiency are potential candidates for repair. However, the success of aortic valve repair is determined largely by the quality of cusp tissue available. Thus, patients with significant leaflet calcification, destruction owing to active endocarditis, or rheumatic involvement are least likely to undergo successful and durable aortic valve repair. In contrast, repair has been shown to have good results in patients with bicuspid (and in smaller series, unicuspid, and quadricuspid aortic valves), despite the abnormalities in cusp anatomy. An important limitation to the universal application of aortic valve repair techniques is the lack of surgical expertise and experience in this field; however, this is changing rapidly with increasing interest in aortic valve repair. Patients who are candidates for repair should be referred to centres with appropriate expertise.

3.13.7.3 Procedures

Surgery of the aortic valve can now be accomplished with greater safety and efficacy in the majority of patients. In patients with higher operative risks, TAVI is already a proven acceptable alternative to AVR. The choice of valve prosthesis is guided by patient preference, life expectancy, and comorbidities relevant to SVD and anticoagulation. Aortic valve repair in the young patient with AR avoids the risks associated with valve prostheses, but long-term durability is unknown. Aortic root surgery similarly can be performed with the replacement of both the aortic valve and aortic wall, but valve-sparing techniques may offer the advantage of durability equivalent to that of normal native aortic valves with avoidance of prosthetic valve-related complications. Reoperative aortic valve and aortic root surgery, like isolated AVR, can be performed safely with best outcomes at high-volume centres.

Aortic valve replacement (AVR) is becoming safe despite the elderly population of patients is now being treated, with the best outcomes achieved at high-volume centres. The standard approach is a median sternotomy aortic valve and aortic root replacement. However, minimally invasive approaches, including the upper hemisternotomy and right anterior thoracotomy (**Figure 4**), can be performed with equivalent safety and better outcomes. The use of stented bioprosthetic valves surpassed the use of mechanical valves, homografts, and pulmonary autografts combined, reflecting advances in valve technology. The Novel Sutureless valves combine the advantages of a surgical AVR procedure (control of aortic atheroemboli, resection of the diseased native valve) with transcatheter technique (decreased procedure time, improved valve hemodynamic function). Bentall procedure: root replacement with a composite valve-graft is the gold standard for aortic root aneurysm (**Figure 5**). However, for patients who want to avoid the long-term oral anticoagulation required for mechanical valves and structural valve deterioration of the bioprosthetic valves, valve-sparing aortic root replacement (David or Yacoub procedures) is a good option (**Figure 6**).

Indications for aortic root replacement include aneurysms of the ascending aorta, aortic valve endocarditis with annular abscess, and acute type A aortic dissection. The most common indication is an aneurysm of the aortic root or ascending aorta. The size threshold for aneurysm repair depends on whether the aneurysm is the primary indication for surgery or whether it coexists in a patient already requiring cardiac surgery.

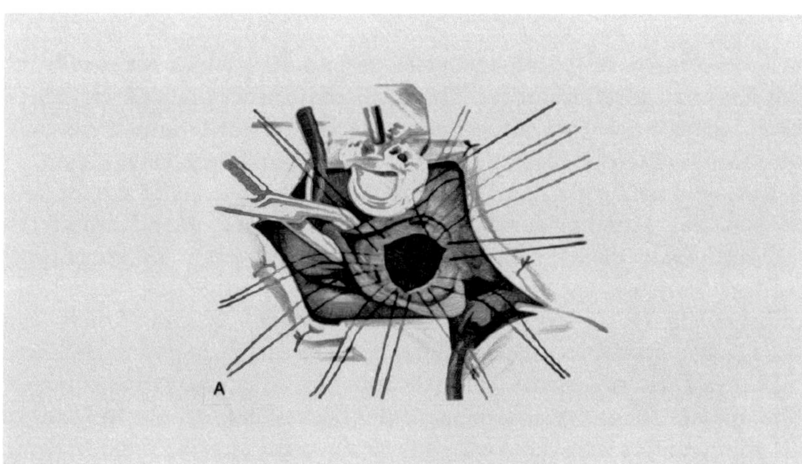

Figure 4.
Aortic valve replacement.

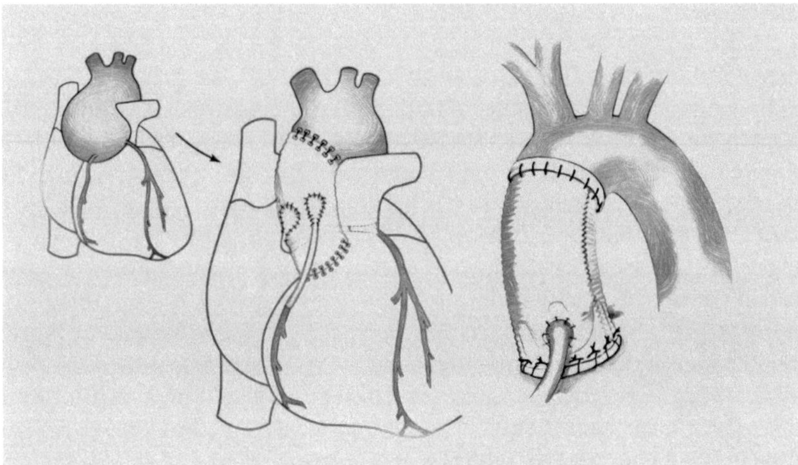

Figure 5.
Bio Bentall procedures.

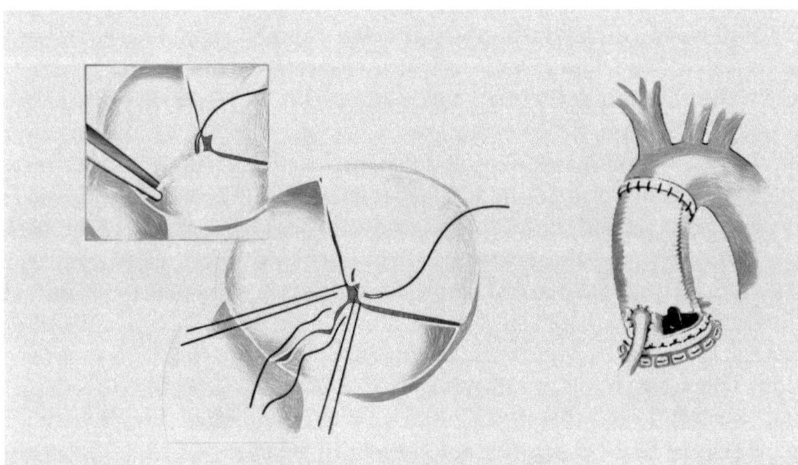

Figure 6.
Valve sparing repair.

Primary aneurysms of the aortic root are secondary to either genetically mediated disorders or acquired disorders. The acquired disorders include degenerative thoracic aortic aneurysm, chronic aortic dissection, intramural hematoma, penetrating atherosclerotic ulcer, mycotic aneurysm, and pseudoaneurysm. The size threshold for surgical repair in this group of patients is 5.5 cm for both the aortic root and ascending aorta according to class I recommendations by the 2010 ACC/AHA Guidelines for the Diagnosis and management of Patients with Thoracic Aortic Disease developed by a multigroup-sponsored task force [65]. The genetically mediated disorders include Marfan syndrome, vascular Ehlers-Danlos syndrome, Turner syndrome, BAV, familial thoracic aortic aneurysm and dissection, and Loeys-Dietz syndrome. These disorders are associated with a greater risk of rupture, dissection, and death, in particular Loeys-Dietz syndrome. The size threshold for operative intervention in this group of patients is 5.0 cm, according to the same guidelines [51]. This recommendation is consistent with a size threshold of 5.0 cm in patients with BAV in the 2006 ACC/AHA Guidelines for the Management of Patients with Valvular Heart Disease [9]. Surgical repair may be considered in patients with Loeys-Dietz syndrome and aortic diameters as small as 4.2 cm, depending on imaging modality [66].

Reoperative aortic valve and aortic root surgery can also be performed safely, utilisation CT/MRI imaging, meticulous myocardial protection, and safe management of existing bypass grafts.

Two devices of aortic valves for percutaneous transcatheter aortic valve implantation (TAVI) have been used in a large number of patients: balloon-expandable and self-expanding. Many new valve technologies are in development [67] (**Figure 7**).

Current data from randomised trials confirmed that TAVI is superior to medical therapy in patients with prohibitive risks for surgery, and it is equivalent to surgical aortic valve replacement in high-risk and medium-risk patients with aortic stenosis [68].

TAVI is technically possible in most patients with aortic stenosis. The larger question is when should TAVI be offered? Evaluation should identify patients in whom a significant improvement in quality and duration of life is likely and avoid unnecessary intervention in patients in whom the procedure can be performed, but the benefit is unlikely. For this reason evaluation of neurocognitive functioning, frailty, functional status, mobility, and social support is important in patient selection [68].

Transthoracic and transesophageal echocardiography, cardiac computed tomography, and invasive angiography are all used to perform anatomic evaluations specific to TAVI.

Evaluation of appropriate candidates for TAVI requires a non-competitive team approach involving interventional cardiologists with expertise in structural heart disease, cardiac and vascular surgeons, anesthesiologists, imaging specialists, and specialised nurses. The proper equipment and a minimum volume of TAVI procedures performed per operator are required.

Randomised trials and large registries of TAVI indicate procedural success rates of more than 95%, 30-day survival of more than 90%, meaningful improvement in the quality of life, and acceptable complication rates (procedure-related stroke < 2%, vascular access site complications < 5%, permanent pacemaker rates < 5%) [69].

Experience with TAVI within failed bioprostheses (valve-in-valve procedures) has been reported. Critical issues in achieving a successful valve-in-valve procedure include an understanding of the manufacturer sizing and labelling of surgical bioprostheses and correct positioning of the valve in the valve. Early experience suggests that TAVI will be an important option for the treatment of patients with failed bioprostheses [70].

More than 100,000 TAVI procedures have been performed to date. Alternatives to TAVI include surgical aortic valve replacement, aortic balloon valvuloplasty (with or without external beam radiation), and apical-to-aortic conduits.

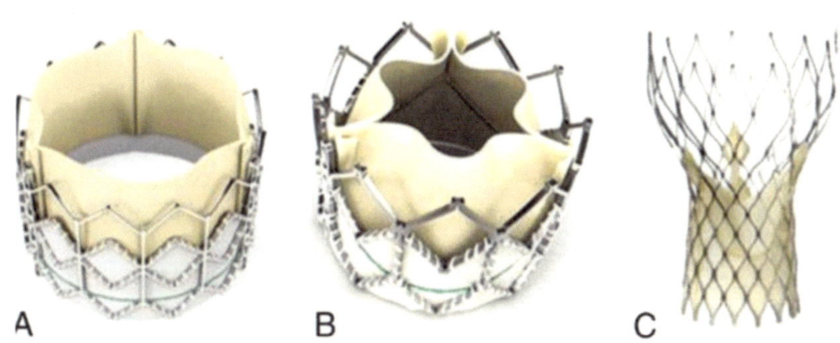

Figure 7.
Current commonly implanted TAVI valves.

3.13.7.4 Outcomes

Data from the STS indicates that the operative mortality for patients 70 years of age or older who underwent isolated AVR or AVR with coronary artery bypass grafting surgery (CABG) between 1994 and 2003 fell from 10% to less than 6% [71]. In the most recent analysis using the STS database on 108,687 patients from 1997 to 2006 with a mean age of 68 years undergoing isolated AVR, the in-hospital mortality was 2.6% with an observed stroke rate of 1.3% and length of stay of 7.8 days for the year 2006. Among patients 80–85 years of age, 30-day mortality was 4.9% with an observed stroke rate of 2.0%.

Experience at centres of excellence within the last 5 years has demonstrated significantly improved operative mortality, less than 1%, after isolated AVR. The incidence of perioperative stroke in these contemporary series ranged from 0% to 1.9%, and the length of stay was as short as 5 days [72].

In the prospective, randomised, multicenter Placement of Aortic Transcatheter Valves (PARTNER) trial comparing high-risk patients (mean STS score 11.8%) receiving TAVI or AVR for severe, symptomatic AS, outcomes for both procedures were excellent [73]. Patients undergoing AVR (n = 351, mean age 85 years) had a 30-day mortality of 6.5%, setting a new benchmark for operative outcomes in a high-risk cohort of patients treated at centres of excellence [74]. Moreover, comparative results showed that early and late strokes and transient ischemic attacks were significantly lower in the AVR group than the TAVI group (30 days, 2.4% vs. 5.5%, respectively, P = 0.04; 1 year, 4.3% vs. 8.3%, respectively, P = 0.04) [75].

Freedom from reoperation depends on both the prosthesis and patient age. Although they do not degenerate, modern mechanical valves do have a finite reoperation rate of 0.5–1% per year from endocarditis, pannus overgrowth, and thrombosis. Actual freedom from reoperation of modern bioprostheses at 15 years approaches 100% in elderly patients older than 70 years, but it can be as low as 50% in patients younger than 50 years.

3.13.7.5 Complications

The most common complications following aortic valve surgery are similar to those of other cardiac surgeries and include stroke (1–4%), deep sternal wound infection (1–2%), reoperation for bleeding (1–3%), and myocardial infarction (MI; 1–5%). Transient heart block is not uncommon, presumably as a result of traction or oedema of the bundle of His in the vicinity of the right noncoronary commissure. It usually resolves within 5–6 days of surgery. The risk of complete heart block requiring pacemaker insertion is 3–5% [76].

4. Summary

Aortic valve replacement is the most commonly performed valve operation. It has been shown to be an effective therapy in all age groups, including the very elderly (age > 90 years). The most common etiologies for AS are calcific degeneration, rheumatic disease, and congenital bicuspid valves. The most common causes of pure aortic regurgitation include annuloaortic ectasia and associated dilation of the aortic root, endocarditis, aortic dissection, and rheumatic disease. The indications for surgery depend on the pathophysiology and symptoms. The choice of the prosthesis can be difficult and depends on multiple clinical and lifestyle considerations. Early and late outcomes are generally quite good, even in high-risk patients.

DOI: http://dx.doi.org/10.5772/intechopen.93311

Author details

Adam El Gamel[1,2,3]

1 Waikato Cardiothoracic Unit, Waikato Hospital, Hamilton, New Zealand

2 Faculty of Medical and Health Sciences, The University of Auckland, Auckland, New Zealand

3 University of Waikato Medical Research Centre, The University of Waikato, New Zealand

*Address all correspondence to: aelgamel@aol.com

References

[1] Filip G, Litwinowicz R, Kapelak B, Sadowski J, Tobota Z, Maruszewski B, et al. Trends in isolated aortic valve replacement in middleaged patients over the last 10 years: Epidemiology, risk factors, valve pathology, valve types, and outcomes. Kardiologia Polska. 2019;**77**:688-695

[2] O'Brien KD. Epidemiology and genetics of calcific aortic valve disease. Journal of Investigative Medicine. 2007;**55**:284-291

[3] Noubiap JJ, Agbor VN, Bigna JJ, Kaze AD, Nyaga UF, Mayosi BM. Prevalence and progression of rheumatic heart disease: A global systematic review and meta-analysis of population-based echocardiographic studies. Scientific Reports. 2019;**9**:17022

[4] Moloi AH, Watkins D, Engel ME, Mall S, Zuhlke L. Epidemiology, health systems and stakeholders in rheumatic heart disease in Africa: A systematic review protocol. BMJ Open. 2016;**6**:e011266

[5] Coffey S, Cox B, Williams MJ. The prevalence, incidence, progression, and risks of aortic valve sclerosis: A systematic review and meta-analysis. Journal of the American College of Cardiology. 2014;**63**:2852-2861

[6] Gaibazzi N, Reverberi C, Ghillani M, Brunazzi B, Faggiano P. Prevalence of undiagnosed asymptomatic aortic valve stenosis in the general population older than 65 years. A screening strategy using cardiac auscultation followed by Doppler-echocardiography. International Journal of Cardiology. 2013;**168**:4905-4906

[7] Osnabrugge RL, Mylotte D, Head SJ, Van Mieghem NM, Nkomo VT, LeReun CM, et al. Aortic stenosis in the elderly: Disease prevalence and number of candidates for transcatheter aortic valve replacement: A meta-analysis and modeling study. Journal of the American College of Cardiology. 2013;**62**:1002-1012

[8] Shah ASV, McAllister DA, Gallacher P, Astengo F, Perez JAR, Hall J, et al. Incidence, microbiology and outcomes in patient hospitalized with infective endocarditis. Circulation. 2020;**141**:2067-2077

[9] Thornhill MH, Dayer MJ, Nicholl J, Prendergast BD, Lockhart PB, Baddour LM. An alarming rise in incidence of infective endocarditis in England since 2009: Why? Lancet. 2020;**395**:1325-1327

[10] Thornhill MH, Gibson TB, Cutler E, Dayer MJ, Chu VH, Lockhart PB, et al. Antibiotic prophylaxis and incidence of endocarditis before and after the 2007 AHA recommendations. Journal of the American College of Cardiology. 2018;**72**:2443-2454

[11] Takkenberg JJ. Biological valves: Is durability really the bottle neck? Heart. 2010;**96**:1691-1692

[12] al-Khaja N, Belboul A, Rashid M, el-Gatit A, Roberts D, Larsson S, et al. The influence of age on the durability of Carpentier-Edwards biological valves. Thirteen years follow-up. European Journal of Cardio-Thoracic Surgery. 1991;**5**:635-640

[13] Terzuolo D. Epidemiology and prophylaxis of the rheumatic fever. Medico-social considerations. Archivio per le Scienze Mediche (Torino). 1968;**125**:391-398

[14] Nagayama T. Social-economic problems of rheumatic fever. Japanese Circulation Journal. 1966;**30**:1339-1340

[15] Cannon JW, Abouzeid M, de Klerk N, Dibben C, Carapetis JR,

Katzenellenbogen JM. Environmental and social determinants of acute rheumatic fever: A longitudinal cohort study. Epidemiology and Infection 2019;**147**:e79

[16] Hashkes PJ. 50 years ago in the journal of pediatrics: Social factors in relation to participation in follow-up care of rheumatic fever. The Journal of Pediatrics. 2013;**162**:535

[17] Kaplan EL, Duckett Jones T. Memorial lecture. Global assessment of rheumatic fever and rheumatic heart disease at the close of the century. Influences and dynamics of populations and pathogens: A failure to realize prevention? Circulation. 1993;**88**:1964-1972

[18] Stollerman GH. Streptococcal vaccines and global strategies for prevention of rheumatic fever. The American Journal of Medicine. 1980;**68**:636-638

[19] Remond MG, Coyle ME, Mills JE, Maguire GP. Approaches to improving adherence to secondary prophylaxis for rheumatic fever and rheumatic heart disease: A literature review with a global perspective. Cardiology in Review. 2016;**24**:94-98

[20] Duchnowski P, Hryniewiecki T, Kusmierczyk M, Szymanski P. The usefulness of selected biomarkers in patients with valve disease. Biomarkers in Medicine. 2018;**12**:1341-1346

[21] Small A, Kiss D, Giri J, Anwaruddin S, Siddiqi H, Guerraty M, et al. Biomarkers of calcific aortic valve disease. Arteriosclerosis, Thrombosis, and Vascular Biology. 2017;**37**:623-632

[22] Moesgaard SG, Falk T, Teerlink T, Guethmundsdottir HH, Sigurethardottir S, Rasmussen CE, et al. Brain-natriuretic peptide and cyclic guanosine monophosphate as biomarkers of myxomatous mitral valve disease in dogs. Veterinary Journal. 2011;**189**:349-352

[23] Christie GW. Anatomy of aortic heart valve leaflets: the influence of glutaraldehyde fixation on function. European Journal of Cardio-Thoracic Surgery. 1992;**6**(Suppl 1):S25-S32

[24] de Kerchove L, Jashari R, Boodhwani M, Duy KT, Lengele B, Gianello P, et al. Surgical anatomy of the aortic root: Implication for valve-sparing reimplantation and aortic valve annuloplasty. The Journal of Thoracic and Cardiovascular Surgery. 2015;**149**:425-433

[25] Rein AJ, Omokhodion SI, Nir A. Significance of a cardiac murmur as the sole clinical sign in the newborn. Clinical Pediatrics (Phila). 2000;**39**:511-520

[26] Shaver JA. Cardiac auscultation: A cost-effective diagnostic skill. Current Problems in Cardiology. 1995;**20**:441-530

[27] Carreras F, Pons-Llado G, Borras X, Padro JM, Caralps JM, Aris A, et al. Non-invasive preoperative assessment of chronic valvular heart disease by Doppler ultrasound. European Heart Journal. 1988;**9**:874-878

[28] Kenny J, Griffin B, McCarthy C, Counihan T. Non-invasive assessment of valvular heart disease using Doppler echocardiography. Irish Medical Journal. 1986;**79**:311-314

[29] Barrett MJ, Lacey CS, Sekara AE, Linden EA, Gracely EJ. Mastering cardiac murmurs: The power of repetition. Chest. 2004;**126**:470-475

[30] Assi ER, Tak T. Assessment of valvular heart disease. Why echocardiography is an essential component. Postgraduate Medical Journal. 1998;**104**:99-102

[31] Chan KL, Stinson WA, Veinot JP. Reliability of transthoracic echocardiography in the assessment of aortic valve morphology: Pathological correlation in

178 patients. The Canadian Journal of Cardiology. 1999;**15**:48-52

[32] Kimura K, Morimoto S. Symptoms and electrocardiographic findings in cardiomyopathies. Nihon Rinsho. 2000;**58**:23-28

[33] Kontogeorgos S, Thunstrom E, Basic C, Hansson PO, Zhong Y, Ergatoudes C, et al. Prevalence and risk factors of aortic stenosis and aortic sclerosis: A 21-year follow-up of middle-aged men. Scandinavian Cardiovascular Journal. 2020;**54**:115-123

[34] Carabello BA. Selection of patients with aortic stenosis for operation: The asymptomatic patient and the patient with poor LV function. Advances in Cardiology. 2002;**39**:49-60

[35] Carabello B. Pathophysiology of valvular heart disease: Implications for nuclear imaging. Journal of Nuclear Cardiology. 2002;**9**:104-113

[36] Zheng KH, Tzolos E, Dweck MR. Pathophysiology of aortic stenosis and future perspectives for medical therapy. Cardiology Clinics. 2020;**38**:1-12

[37] Thrasher JR, Talley JD. Syncope and aortic valve stenosis: Clues to diagnosis and pathophysiology. The Journal of the Arkansas Medical Society. 1996;**93**:191-193

[38] Ross J Jr, Braunwald E. Aortic stenosis. Circulation. 1968;**38**:61-67

[39] Bhattacharyya S, Mittal T, Abayalingam M, Kabir T, Dalby M, Cleland JG, et al. Classification of aortic stenosis by flow and gradient patterns provides insights into the pathophysiology of disease. Angiology. 2016;**67**:664-669

[40] Braunwald E. On the natural history of severe aortic stenosis. Journal of the American College of Cardiology. 1990;**15**:1018-1020

[41] Lee HJ, Kim HK. Natural history data in symptomatic severe aortic stenosis alerts cardiologists to the dangers of no action. Korean Circulation Journal. 2019;**49**:170-172

[42] Herrmann S, Fries B, Liu D, Hu K, Stoerk S, Voelker W, et al. Differences in natural history of low- and high-gradient aortic stenosis from nonsevere to severe stage of the disease. Journal of the American Society of Echocardiography. 2015;**28**:1270-1282

[43] Ishii K, Hirota Y, Suwa M, Kita Y, Onaka H, Kawamura K. Natural history and left ventricular response in chronic aortic regurgitation. The American Journal of Cardiology. 1996;**78**:357-361

[44] Dervan J, Goldberg S. Acute aortic regurgitation: Pathophysiology and management. Cardiovascular Clinics. 1986;**16**:281-288

[45] Pisacane C, Pacileo G, Santoro G, Sarubbi B, Iacono C, Russo MG, et al. New insights in the pathophysiology of mitral and aortic regurgitation in pediatric age: Role of angiotensin-converting enzyme inhibitor therapy. Italian Heart Journal. 2001;**2**:100-106

[46] Shigenobu M, Sano S. The clinical and pathological features of isolated aortic regurgitation in relation to its etiology. Surgery Today. 1994;**24**:393-398

[47] Lancellotti P, Rosenhek R, Pibarot P, Iung B, Otto CM, Tornos P, et al. ESC working group on valvular heart disease position paper—Heart valve clinics: Organization, structure, and experiences. European Heart Journal. 2013;**34**:1597-1606

[48] Markowitz M, Gerber MA. The Jones criteria for guidance in the diagnosis of rheumatic fever. Another perspective. Archives of Pediatrics & Adolescent Medicine. 1995;**149**:725-726

[49] Shulman ST, Amren DP, Bisno AL, Dajani AS, Durack DT, Gerber MA, et al. Prevention of rheumatic fever. A statement for health professionals by the committee on rheumatic fever and infective endocarditis of the council on cardiovascular disease in the young. Circulation. 1984;**70**:1118A-1122A

[50] Wilson W, Taubert KA, Gewitz M, Lockhart PB, Baddour LM, Levison M, et al. Prevention of infective endocarditis: Guidelines from the American Heart Association: A guideline from the American Heart Association Rheumatic Fever, Endocarditis and Kawasaki Disease Committee, Council on Cardiovascular Disease in the Young, and the Council on Clinical Cardiology, Council on Cardiovascular Surgery and Anesthesia, and the Quality of Care and Outcomes Research Interdisciplinary Working Group. Journal of the American Dental Association. 2008;**139**(Suppl):3S-24S

[51] Whitlock RP, Sun JC, Fremes SE, Rubens FD, Teoh KH. Antithrombotic and thrombolytic therapy for valvular disease: Antithrombotic therapy and prevention of thrombosis, 9th ed: American College of Chest Physicians Evidence-Based Clinical Practice Guidelines. Chest. 2012;**141**:e576S-e600S

[52] Whitlock RP, Eikelboom JW. Prevention of thromboembolic events after bioprosthetic aortic valve replacement: What is the optimal antithrombotic strategy? Journal of the American College of Cardiology. 2012;**60**:978-980

[53] Fuster V, Ryden LE, Cannom DS, Crijns HJ, Curtis AB, Ellenbogen KA, et al. ACCF/AHA/HRS focused updates incorporated into the ACC/AHA/ESC 2006 Guidelines for the management of patients with atrial fibrillation: A report of the American College of Cardiology Foundation/American Heart Association Task Force on Practice Guidelines developed in partnership with the European Society of Cardiology and in collaboration with the European Heart Rhythm Association and the Heart Rhythm Society. Journal of the American College of Cardiology. 2011;**57**:e101-e198

[54] Fleisher LA, Beckman JA, Brown KA, Calkins H, Chaikof E, Fleischmann KE, et al. ACC/AHA 2006 guideline update on perioperative cardiovascular evaluation for noncardiac surgery: Focused update on perioperative beta-blocker therapy: A report of the American College of Cardiology/American Heart Association task force on practice guidelines (writing committee to update the 2002 guidelines on perioperative cardiovascular evaluation for noncardiac surgery): Developed in collaboration with the American Society of Echocardiography, American Society of Nuclear Cardiology, Heart Rhythm Society, Society of Cardiovascular Anesthesiologists, Society for Cardiovascular Angiography and Interventions, and Society for Vascular Medicine and Biology. Circulation. 2006;**113**:2662-2674

[55] Michalski B, Dweck MR, Marsan NA, Cameli M, D'Andrea A, Carvalho RF, et al. The evaluation of aortic stenosis, how the new guidelines are implemented across Europe: A survey by EACVI. European Heart Journal Cardiovascular Imaging. 2020;**21**:357-362

[56] Kolkailah AA, Doukky R, Pelletier MP, Volgman AS, Kaneko T, Nabhan AF. Cochrane corner: Trans-catheter aortic valve implantation versus surgical aortic valve replacement for severe aortic stenosis in people with low surgical risk. Heart. Cochrane Database of Systematic Reviews. John Wiley & Sons, Ltd; 2019. Issue No. 12. SN: 1465-1858

[57] Kanwar A, Thaden JJ, Nkomo VT. Management of patients with aortic

valve stenosis. Mayo Clinic Proceedings. 2018;**93**:488-508

[58] Harris AW, Pibarot P, Otto CM. Aortic stenosis: Guidelines and evidence gaps. Cardiology Clinics. 2020;**38**:55-63

[59] Malik AH, Zaid S, Ahmad H, Goldberg J, Dutta T, Undemir C, et al. A meta-analysis of 1-year outcomes of transcatheter versus surgical aortic valve replacement in low-risk patients with severe aortic stenosis. Journal of Geriatric Cardiology. 2020;**17**:43-50

[60] Monin JL, Quere JP, Monchi M, Petit H, Baleynaud S, Chauvel C, et al. Low-gradient aortic stenosis: Operative risk stratification and predictors for long-term outcome: A multicenter study using dobutamine stress hemodynamics. Circulation. 2003;**108**:319-324

[61] Yoon SH, Schmidt T, Bleiziffer S, Schofer N, Fiorina C, Munoz-Garcia AJ, et al. Transcatheter aortic valve replacement in pure native aortic valve regurgitation. Journal of the American College of Cardiology. 2017;**70**:2752-2763

[62] Bando K. Filling the gap between guidelines and current surgical practice: Is early surgery justified in patients with asymptomatic severe aortic regurgitation with normal left ventricular function? Seminars in Thoracic and Cardiovascular Surgery. 2019;**31**:771-772

[63] Yang LT, Michelena HI, Scott CG, Enriquez-Sarano M, Pislaru SV, Schaff HV, et al. Outcomes in chronic hemodynamically significant aortic regurgitation and limitations of current guidelines. Journal of the American College of Cardiology. 2019;**73**:1741-1752

[64] David TE, Feindel CM. An aortic valve-sparing operation for patients with aortic incompetence and aneurysm of the ascending aorta. The Journal of Thoracic and Cardiovascular Surgery. 1992;**103**:617-621

[65] Milewicz DM, Regalado ES, Guo DC. Treatment guidelines for thoracic aortic aneurysms and dissections based on the underlying causative gene. The Journal of Thoracic and Cardiovascular Surgery. 2010;**140**:S2-S4

[66] Cooper MA, Upchurch GR Jr. The society of vascular surgery practice guidelines on the care of patients with abdominal aortic aneurysms. JAMA Surgery. 2019;**154**:553-554

[67] Scherman J, Weich H. SASCI/SCTSSA joint consensus statement and guidelines on transcatheter aortic valve implantation (TAVI) in South Africa. Cardiovascular Journal of Africa. 2016;**27**:399-400

[68] Lung B. Aortic stenosis in the elderly: Surgery or TAVI. New European guidelines. Presse Médicale. 2013;**42**:986-994

[69] Pighi M, Serdoz R, Kilic ID, Sherif SA, Lindsay A, Di Mario C. TAVI: New trials and registries offer further welcome evidence—U.S. CoreValve, CHOICE, and GARY. Global Cardiology Science and Practice. 2014;**2014**:78-87

[70] Giordana F, Bruno F, Conrotto F, Saglietto A, D'Ascenzo F, Marra WG, et al. Incidence, predictors and outcomes of valve-in-valve TAVI: A systematic review and meta-analysis. International Journal of Cardiology. 2020;**316**(2020):64-69

[71] Ram E, Amunts S, Zuroff E, Peled Y, Kogan A, Raanani E, et al. Outcomes of isolated surgical aortic valve replacement in the era of transcatheter aortic valve implantation. Journal of Cardiac Surgery. 20 July 2020;**35**(7):1395-1748

[72] Mazine A, El-Hamamsy I. Procedures and outcomes of surgical aortic valve replacement in adults. Cardiology Clinics. 2020;**38**:89-102

[73] Mack MJ, Leon MB, Smith CR, Miller DC, Moses JW, Tuzcu EM, et al. 5-Year outcomes of transcatheter aortic valve replacement or surgical aortic valve replacement for high surgical risk patients with aortic stenosis (PARTNER 1): A randomised controlled trial. Lancet. 2015;**385**:2477-2484

[74] Tang GH, Lansman SL, Panza JA. Beyond PARTNER: Appraising the evolving trends and outcomes in transcatheter aortic valve replacement. Cardiology in Review. 2015;**23**:1-10

[75] Thourani VH, Jensen HA, Babaliaros V, Kodali SK, Rajeswaran J, Ehrlinger J, et al. Outcomes in nonagenarians undergoing transcatheter aortic valve replacement in the PARTNER-I trial. Annals of Thoracic Surgery. 2015;**100**:785-792

[76] Tamburino C, Barbanti M, Capodanno D, Mignosa C, Gentile M, Aruta P, et al. Comparison of complications and outcomes to one year of transcatheter aortic valve implantation versus surgical aortic valve replacement in patients with severe aortic stenosis. The American Journal of Cardiology. 2012;**109**:1487-1493

Chapter 3

Clinical Applications of Strain Imaging in Aortic Valve Disease

Ernesto E. Salcedo and Edward A. Gill

Abstract

The prevalence of aortic valve disease, particularly aortic stenosis, is increasing in parallel to the aging of the population, making it the most prevalent form of valvular heart disease. Surgery and percutaneous interventions of the aortic valve are conditional to a comprehensive evaluation of the aortic valve and the left ventricle (LV). Favorable results from aortic valve surgery or intervention are influenced by LV ejection fraction (EF), presence and severity of left ventricular hypertrophy (LVH), LV end-systolic volume (LVESV), degree of leaflet calcification, and trans-aortic valve gradients. Deformation imaging, particularly global longitudinal strain, is evolving as a powerful tool in the evaluation of ventricular function in patients with aortic stenosis. GLS is particularly suited to detect subclinical LV dysfunction, before a drop in LV ejection fraction, providing the opportunity to intervene earlier to prevent serious and permanent LV dysfunction. Similar added value has been demonstrated in the application of GLS in the detection of subclinical LV dysfunction in patients with aortic regurgitation. Very little information exists in the use of GLS in patients with mixed aortic valve disease, providing an opportunity for future research in this important group of patients with aortic valve disease.

Keywords: aortic stenosis, aortic regurgitation, aortic valve surgery, aortic valve intervention, global longitudinal strain

1. Introduction

As the population grows older, the prevalence of aortic valve disease, particularly aortic stenosis, is swelling, making it currently, the most prevalent form of valvular heart disease [1–3]. Surgery and percutaneous interventions of the aortic valve are frequently needed in patients with severe symptomatic aortic valve disease, the timing for these procedures' conditional on a comprehensive evaluation of the dysfunctional aortic valve and the resultant repercussions on the rest of the heart, particularly the left ventricle (LV). Parameters used to predict favorable/unfavorable results from aortic valve surgery or intervention include LV ejection fraction (EF), presence and severity of left ventricular hypertrophy

IntechOpen

(LVH), LV end-systolic volume (LVESV), degree of leaflet calcification, and trans-aortic valve gradients. Because of the LV deformation indices potential to detect subclinical LV dysfunction, they are being used with increasing frequency in the management of patients with aortic valve disease [4] and advancing the timing for aortic valve surgery or intervention, before the LV is irreversibly damaged.

Our objective with this chapter is to describe the use of strain imaging, particularly global longitudinal strain in the assessment of cardiac function in patients with aortic valve disease. We review the current clinical applications of strain analysis in patients with aortic valve disease, highlighting strengths and weaknesses and emphasizing normal and abnormal findings in aortic stenosis (AS) aortic regurgitation (AR) and mixed aortic valve disease (ASAR); we summarize unresolved issues, potential future research priorities, and recommended indications for incorporating this technique into the clinical practice of patients with aortic valve disease.

2. Strain imaging: general principles

Strain is defined as the fractional change in length of a myocardial segment relative to its baseline length, it is expressed as a percentage. Strain rate is the temporal derivative of strain, providing information on the speed at which the deformation occurs. Echocardiography, because of its dynamic nature, is ideally suited for the evaluation of cardiac mechanics through the application of deformation indices [5, 6]. Two echocardiographic techniques have dominated the clinical and research arena of deformation echocardiography: (1) tissue Doppler imaging, and (2) speckle tracking imaging. Both techniques lend to the derivation of multiple parameters of myocardial function. Tissue Doppler Imaging (TDI) was the first method used to measure myocardial deformation by echocardiography. The method is well validated and has been shown to provide valuable data in a wide range of conditions. Tissue Doppler is currently used mainly for evaluation of diastolic LV function, its use in aortic valve disease will not be discussed in this chapter. Speckle tracking, mainly through the use of global longitudinal strain (GLS), is increasingly used to identify subclinical myocardial dysfunction in patients with valvular heart disease and to identify optimal timing for surgery or intervention and prognosticate outcomes after surgery/intervention, and is the main focus of this review.

3. Strain imaging in aortic stenosis

Aortic stenosis inflicts progressive pressure overload on the LV with compensatory concentric hypertrophy (**Figure 1**). Initially, the increased wall thickness and conservation of normal LV chamber dimensions offsets the increased LV pressure, maintaining a normal ejection fraction. If the aortic stenosis is not corrected it will inexorably lead to reduced myocardial perfusion, and eventual fibrosis with consequent drop in ejection fraction. It is well recognized that LV GLS is superior to LVEF in detecting perturbations in myocardial function. Compared with normal controls, severe aortic stenosis patients have impaired strain in all three layers of the LV myocardium. LV strain analysis in aortic stenosis has been evaluated in different settings as noted in the following sections.

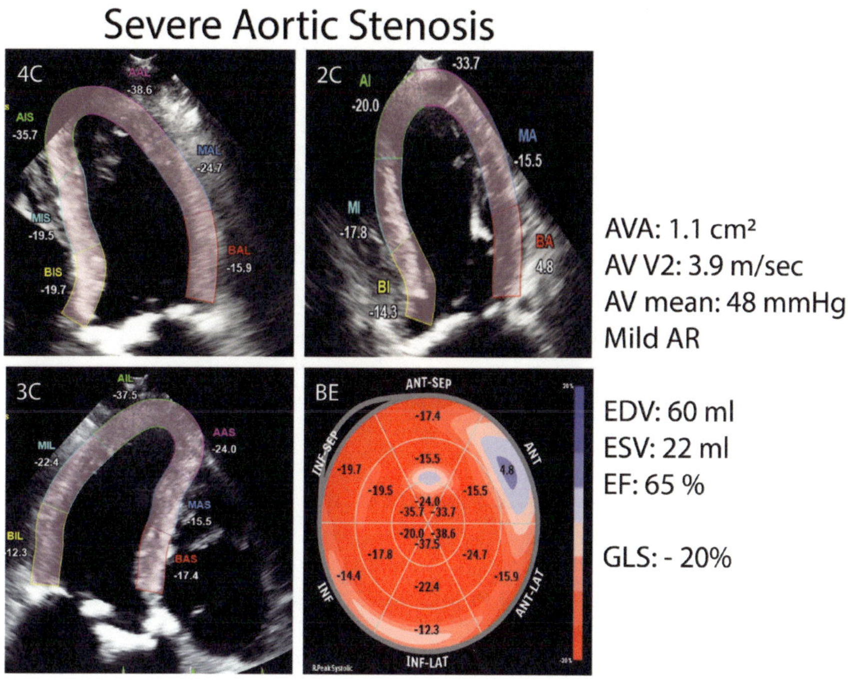

Figure 1.
Severe aortic stenosis: global longitudinal strain (GLS) in a patient with severe aortic stenosis with an aortic valve area (AVA) of 1.1 cm² maximal velocity (AV V2) of 3.9 m/s and a mean gradient of 48 mm Hg. Left ventricular end-diastolic and end-systolic volumes (EDV, ESV) are normal as well as the LV ejection fraction (EF). The GLS is normal at −20% indicating absence of any LV dysfunction.

4. Strain imaging and ejection fraction in aortic stenosis

Measuring LV ejection fraction is crucial in the management of patients with asymptomatic severe aortic stenosis (AS). According to the current American Heart Association/American College of Cardiology and European Society of Cardiology guidelines there is a Class I indication (Level of Evidence: B) to perform aortic valve intervention in asymptomatic patients with severe AS when the LVEF becomes <50% [7, 8]. Predictors of poor outcome in aortic stenosis include advanced age, significant leaflet calcification, rapid disease progression and decreased left ventricular (LV) ejection fraction (EF). Patients can develop impaired LVEF due to afterload mismatch or from true depression of myocardial contractility due to myocardial fibrosis. Myocardial fibrosis occurs early in the natural history of aortic stenosis, affecting diastolic and systolic function and offering a substrate for ventricular arrhythmias, playing a role in the progression to heart failure and sudden cardiac death. These observations indicate that current echocardiographic assessment of LV function by measuring only the LVEF is insufficient and that new parameters detecting subtle myocardial impairment are needed to improve risk stratification and predict outcomes in patients with AS.

Several studies have defined the added value of global longitudinal strain over LVEF to characterize and prognosticate the clinical evolution of patients with aortic stenosis:

- There is growing evidence suggesting the prognostic role of global longitudinal strain (GLS), in asymptomatic patients with AS. The American Society of

Echocardiography (ASE) on cardiac chamber quantification acknowledged the incremental value of LV GLS over traditional LVEF measurements, and recommended its clinical use in patients [9].

- Conventional measures of LVEF can be preserved until end-stage disease due to the compensatory development of concentric hypertrophy, and thus lacks accuracy in identifying subtle changes in myocardial contractility [2].

- Subclinical myocardial dysfunction with impaired LV GLS is frequently seen in patients with severe AS with preserved LVEF and no symptoms. Left ventricular global longitudinal strain deteriorates over time and impaired LV GLS at baseline is associated with an increased risk for progression to the symptomatic stage and the need for aortic valve surgery or intervention [10].

5. Strain imaging and aortic stenosis severity

A relationship between aortic stenosis severity and alterations in LV deformation indices has been demonstrated in the following studies:

- Strain and strain rate parameters relate to LV function and aortic stenosis severity. Further, they appear to be superior to tissue velocity and conventional echocardiography in detecting subtle changes in myocardial function after AVR before LV mass and LV function show improvement [11].

- Despite unchanged LVEF, GLS gradually decreased as severity of AS increases. GLS measured by 2D-speckle tracking imaging might be useful to assess subtle changes in LV function in AS patients [12].

6. Strain imaging—prognostic value in aortic stenosis

LV strain analysis has been demonstrated to provide prognostic information in patients with aortic stenosis:

- A recent met analysis, including 1067 asymptomatic patients, with AS and preserved LVEF, showed that LVGLS is strongly associated with mortality, with >2.5-fold increase in risk of death in patients with impaired LVGLS (−14.7% or less) [13].

- GLS detects subclinical dysfunction and has incremental prognostic value over traditional risk markers including hemodynamic severity, symptom class, and LVEF in patients with AS. Incorporation of GLS into risk models can improve the identification of the optimal timing for AV replacement [14].

- Kusunose et al. [15] demonstrated on 395 patients that Longitudinal strain (LS) is independently associated with death in patients with AS and preserved LVEF, in addition they made the point that the flow/gradient pattern should also be considered as an important parameter. In the management of AS patients the use apical 4 chamber LS should be considered a new parameter of evaluation of LV function and prognosis [16].

- LV GLS is independently associated with all-cause mortality in AS patients. It can further risk stratify severe AS patients and may influence the optimal timing of aortic valve replacement [2].

- GLS is an independent predictor of all-cause mortality in severe AS, irrespective of their type of treatment. GLS <9.7% indicates a significantly higher 1- and 5-year mortality in non-AVR patients. Therefore, GLS should be regularly assessed for enhanced risk stratification and clinical decision-making [17].

- In normal LVEF patients with significant aortic stenosis, brain natriuretic peptide (BNP) and LV-GLS provide incremental prognostic information over established predictors, suggesting that both play a synergistic role in defining outcomes [18].

- A drop in LVGLS in bicuspid aortic valve (BAV) with preserved LVEF is not infrequent and was independently associated with increased risk of events (mainly aortic valve replacement events), as found by Kong et al. [19] in 513 patients (68% men; mean age 44 ± 18 years) with BAV and preserved LVEF (>50%).

7. Strain imaging in combined aortic stenosis and coronary artery disease

Subclinical coronary artery disease is common in moderate and severe aortic stenosis, and should be suspected when regional longitudinal dysfunction is predominant in the apical and mid ventricular segments [20].

8. Strain imaging sublayers in aortic stenosis

Sublayer strain analysis may add additional information in the characterization of LV function in patients with aortic stenosis. The following studies address this issue:

- In severe AS, longitudinal strain impairment affects all three myocardial layers but is more noticeable in the endocardial layer. This becomes more manifest in the advanced phases of the disease when symptoms appear [21].

- Bilayer strain ratio (subendocardial and subepicardial) can reliably differentiate patients with varying degrees of AS severity and is a sensitive marker of LV function. These findings suggest that the evaluation of subendocardial and subepicardial radial strain might be a novel method for assessing LV mechanics in patients with AS [22].

- Medically treated patients with AS have worsening of GLS despite preserved LVEF, first appearing in the subendocardial layer. Global circumferential strain (GCS) becomes progressively impaired in moderate and severe AS. Improvement in LV strain after AVR is seen earlier with GLS than with GCS [23].

- There is differential impairment in LV systolic strain in all three cardiac axes in patients with AS. Left ventricular longitudinal strain impairment is proportional to AS severity. Subendocardial longitudinal strain correlates better with

AS severity than subepicardial longitudinal strain while correlations between circumferential and radial strain and AS severity are weak [24].

- Compared with normal controls, severe aortic stenosis patients have impaired strain in all three layers of the LV myocardium [25].

9. Strain imaging in low gradient severe aortic stenosis

Several studies have characterized the LV deformation indices in patients with low gradient aortic stenosis:

- GLS is depressed in patients with paradoxic low flow (PLF) AS. This implies that subclinical myocardial dysfunction may be more prominent in PLF AS compared with normal-flow AS and suggests the possible diagnostic and prognostic value of two-dimensional global strain in identifying PLF AS [26].

- In patients with low flow-low gradient aortic stenosis, 2-dimensional strain parameters are strong predictors of outcome. Peak longitudinal strain rate may add incremental prognostic value beyond what is obtained from N-terminal pro-B-type natriuretic peptide and peak stress left ventricular ejection fraction [27].

- Sato et al. [28] demonstrated in 204 patients that longitudinal LV function is severely impaired in patients with paradoxical low-flow, low-gradient (LFLPG) AS and they have a poor prognosis. GLS could stratify the high-risk group for future adverse outcomes.

- Patients with paradoxical low-flow severe aortic stenosis (PLF-AS) reportedly have higher left ventricular hydraulic load and more systolic strain dysfunction than patients with normal-flow aortic stenosis. Holmes et al. [29] investigated the relationship of systolic loading and strain to PLF-AS in 120 patients. Patients with PLF-AS were found to have more valvular load, lower energy loss coefficient, more arterial load and increased systemic vascular resistance and more total hydraulic load. They concluded that Increased hydraulic load, from more severe valvular stenosis and increased vascular resistance, and longitudinal strain impairment are associated with PLF-AS and their interplay is likely fundamental to its pathophysiology.

- Dahou et al. [30] examined the impact of left ventricular (LV) global longitudinal strain (GLS) measured at rest and at dobutamine stress echocardiography on the outcome of 202 patients with low LV ejection fraction and low-gradient aortic stenosis. GLS was found to be independently associated with mortality in patients with low LV ejection fraction, low-gradient aortic stenosis. Stress GLS measured during dobutamine stress echocardiography provided incremental prognostic value beyond GLS measured at rest in these patients. Hence, these authors concluded that measurement of GLS at rest and during dobutamine stress echocardiography may be helpful to enhance risk stratification in low LV ejection fraction, low-gradient aortic stenosis.

- In patients with LF-LG AS and low LVEF, reduced right ventricular longitudinal strain (RVLS) was found by Dahou et al. [31] to be independently associated with increased risk of mortality. Furthermore, stress RVLS provided incremental prognostic value beyond that obtained from rest RVLS. Thus, RVLS measurement at rest and with dobutamine stress may be helpful to enhance risk stratification in this high-risk population.

10. Strain imaging in aortic stenosis—effects of hypertension

The added effect of hypertension in deformation indices abnormalities has been defined in the following studies:

- Hypertension has significant negative effect on LV mechanics in patients with aortic stenosis. Blood pressure is associated with deterioration of LV global longitudinal and circumferential strains in aortic stenosis patients independently of clinical and demographic characteristics [32].

- In AS, both the AS severity and concomitant hypertension attenuate radial tissue Doppler imaging strain in the inferior LV wall. The subendocardial radial strain is mainly influenced by AS severity, while midmyocardial radial strain is attenuated by both hypertension and AS severity [33].

11. Strain imaging and aortic valve surgery/intervention

The contributions of LV strain analysis in the surgical or interventional management of patients with aortic stenosis has been extensively documented. The following statements summarize the conclusions of several studies addressing the use of strain imaging as it relates to valve replacement or intervention in patients with aortic stenosis.

- LV longitudinal systolic strain is depressed despite preserved LV ejection fraction and fractional shortening in AS. A significant association exists among natriuretic peptides, myocardial longitudinal contractility, and the degree of symptoms. Reverse LV remodeling after aortic valve replacement with regression of myocardial hypertrophy results in improvement of LV longitudinal myocardial strain and decrease of Nt-pro-BNP plasma levels. LV strain analysis has the potential to identify patients with asymptomatic AS who might benefit from earlier surgical intervention to preserve overall LV function [34].

- In patients with symptomatic severe aortic stenosis undergoing aortic valve replacement, reduced GLS (Particularly in the setting of normal LVEF) provides important prognostic information beyond standard risk factors [35].

- Shortly after balloon valvuloplasty for severe congenital AS, there is an improvement in systolic myocardial deformation. However, two-dimensional speckle-tracking echocardiographic parameters do not return to normal at 3-year follow-up. These abnormalities in systolic deformation cannot be fully attributed to residual stenosis or aortic regurgitation [36].

- Marcus et al. [36] showed in 37 children that shortly after balloon valvuloplasty for severe congenital AS, there is an improvement in systolic myocardial deformation. However, two-dimensional speckle tracking echocardiography parameters do not return to normal at 3-year follow-up. These abnormalities in systolic deformation cannot be fully attributed to residual stenosis or aortic regurgitation.

- Kafa et al. [37] evaluated 208 patients that underwent AVR for severe AS, measuring GLS pre and 12–24 months post AVR and found that in patients with severe aortic stenosis, approximately 20% of patients who survived more than 1 year after aortic valve replacement had an abnormal LV-GLS value on postoperative echocardiography, despite a preserved postoperative LVEF and demonstrable left ventricular mass regression. This finding was independently associated with adverse events, concluding that appropriately timed aortic valve replacement relieves left ventricular wall stress and prevents a decline in LVEF.

- In asymptomatic/minimally symptomatic patients with severe bioprosthetic AS undergoing redo aortic valve replacement (AVR), baseline LV-GLS provides incremental prognostic value over established predictors and could potentially aid in surgical timing and risk stratification [38].

- AVR reverses LA abnormalities and regains normal atrial function, a behavior which is directly related to the severity of preoperative LV outflow tract obstruction. Early identification of LA size enlargement and functional disturbances might contribute to better patient's recruitment for AVR [39].

- Speckle echocardiography analysis of left atrial (LA) myocardial deformation is considered a promising tool for the evaluation of LA subclinical dysfunction in patients undergoing AVR, giving a potentially better risk stratification for the occurrence of postoperative atrial fibrillation [40].

- Gelsomino et al. [41] explored the influence of global longitudinal strain measured with two-dimensional speckle-tracking echocardiography on left ventricular mass regression (LVMR) in 83 patients with pure aortic stenosis (AS) and normal left ventricular function undergoing aortic valve replacement (AVR) and found that global longitudinal strain accurately predicts LV mass regression in patients with pure AS undergoing AVR.

In summary LV GLS can detect subclinical myocardial dysfunction in patients with severe aortic stenosis, and progressively worsens with increasing aortic stenosis severity. Impaired LV GLS is independently associated with increased mortality in high-gradient aortic stenosis, in low-flow, low-gradient severe aortic stenosis with preserved LVEF, and in low-flow, low-gradient severe aortic stenosis with reduced LVEF. Strain analysis of specific myocardial sublayers may add value to the evaluation of strain in aortic stenosis. Coronary artery disease and hypertension produce additional variables in strain analysis that need to be considered. Finally, there is increasing support for the use of strain imaging to determine the need and timing for aortic valve surgery or intervention in patients with aortic stenosis.

12. Strain imaging in aortic regurgitation

In contrast to aortic stenosis, aortic regurgitation (AR) generates LV volume overload with progressive LV dilatation, initially with preservation of LVEF and wall thickness (eccentric LV hypertrophy), but eventually with the development of LV systolic dysfunction expressed by a drop in LVEF (**Figure 2**). Several studies have described the value of strain imaging in the management of patients with aortic regurgitation. The results and conclusion statement of these studies are summarized in the following paragraphs:

- In patient with AR, LV strain analysis can detect early subclinical myocardial dysfunction before the development of impaired LVEF. Using tissue Doppler imaging, Marciniak et al. [42] demonstrated that patients with severe AR had significant impairment of LV longitudinal strain, in contrast to patients with moderate AR where there was no difference with controls.

- Smedsrud et al. [43] evaluated 47 AR patients and 31 controls with Longitudinal peak systolic strain rate and found they were significantly decreased in the patient's population ($P < 0.001$). Global longitudinal peak systolic strain rate was also significantly decreased in aortic stenosis and regurgitation compared to the control group (-1 ± 0.5, -0.9 ± 0.3, and -1.6 ± 0.3, $P = 0.001$). As far as the comparison between patients with aortic stenosis and aortic regurgitation, neither global strain rate nor strain rate for each wall was found to be different. They concluded that there was reduced global longitudinal strain in patients with chronic AR with preserved LV ejection fractions. Global longitudinal strain might therefore disclose incipient myocardial dysfunction with a consequent potential for improved timing of aortic valve surgery.

- Di Salvo et al. [44] evaluated 26 young patients (3-16 years) with asymptomatic AR and found LV average longitudinal strain to be significantly reduced in patients with progressive AR compared to those with stable AR ($-17.8 \pm 3.9\%$ vs. $-22.7 \pm 2.7\%$, $p = 0.001$). On multivariate analysis, the only significant risk factor for progressive AR was average LV longitudinal strain ($p = 0.04$, cut-off value $> -19.5\%$, sensitivity 77.8%, specificity 94.1%, area under the curve 0.889). These authors concluded that two-dimensional strain imaging

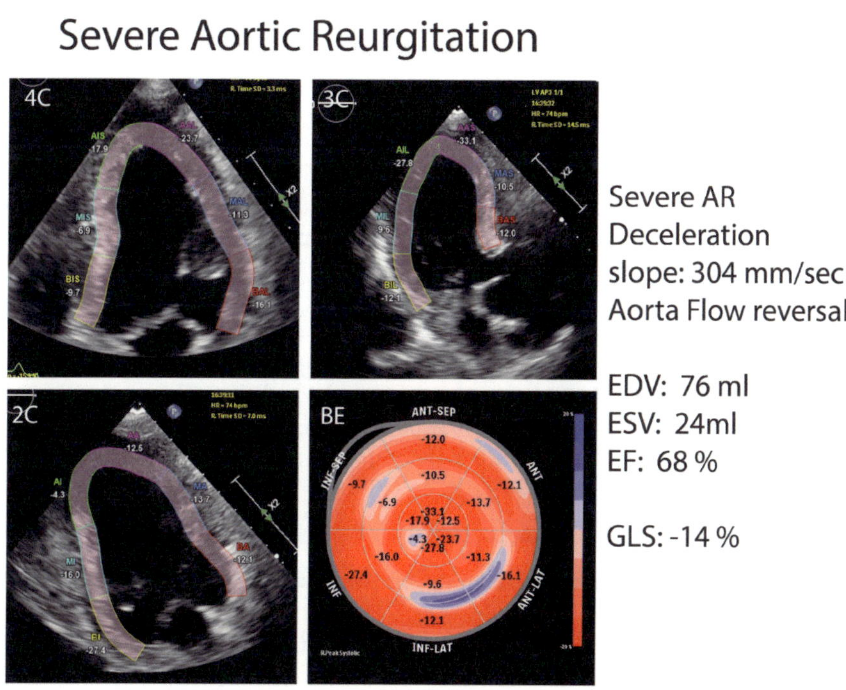

Figure 2.
Severe aortic regurgitation: this patient had severe aortic regurgitation with normal LV end-diastolic and end-systolic volumes (EDV, ESV) and preserved systolic function as estimated by a normal LV ejection fraction (EF) of 68%; however, there is already evidence of insipient LV dysfunction as demonstrated by a mild drop in global longitudinal strain at –14%.

can discriminate young asymptomatic patients with progressive AR. This could allow young patients with AR to have a better definition of surgical timing before the occurrence of irreversible myocardial damage.

- Kaneko et al. [45] evaluated 36 chronic AR patients undergoing surgical correction and found, with the use of speckle-tracking strain imaging, that LV subendocardial dysfunction was present in patients with chronic severe AR and preserved EF, this improved after surgical correction.

- Park et al. [46] evaluated 60 patients with chronic AR with LV global strain rate on apical four chamber image (GS-4CH). During 64 months follow-up duration, 16 patients (26.7%) were deceased and 38 patients (63.3%) underwent aortic valve replacement (AVR). Deceased group had lower longitudinal strain (−12.05 ± 3.72% vs. -15.66 ± 4.35%, $p = 0.005$). On multivariate analysis by cox proportional hazard model adjusting for age, sex, body surface area, history of atrial fibrillation, blood urea nitrogen, LV dilatation, LV ejection fraction and AVR, decreased GS-4CH proved to be an independent predictor of mortality in patients with chronic AR (hazard ratio 1.313, 95% confidence interval 1.010–1.706, $p = 0.042$). They concluded that GS-4CH may be a useful predictor of mortality in patient with chronic AR.

- Alashi et al. [47] evaluated 1063 patients with asymptomatic severe chronic AR and preserved LVEF to examine the prognostic utility of left ventricular (LV) global longitudinal strain (GLS). A significantly higher proportion (log-rank $p = 0.01$) of patients with LV-GLS worse than median (−19.5%) died versus those with an LV-GLS better than median [86 of 513 (17%) vs. 60 of 550 (11%)]. The risk of death at 5 years significantly increased with an LV-GLS of worse than −19%. They concluded that in asymptomatic patients with ≥III+ chronic AR and preserved LVEF, worsening LV-GLS was associated with longer term mortality, providing incremental prognostic value and improved reclassification.

- Alashi et al. [48] evaluated 865 patients with ≥3+ chronic AR and preserved LVEF undergoing AV surgery, a baseline LV-GLS value worse than −19% was associated with reduced survival. In a subgroup of patients who returned for 3- and 12-month postoperative follow-up examinations, persistently impaired LV-GLS was associated with increased mortality.

In summary, in patients with severe AR LV strain analysis detects early subclinical myocardial. Dysfunction before there is a drop in LVEF. This provides the potential for improving AVR/intervention timing. In addition GLS may be a useful predictor of mortality in AR patients by providing incremental prognostic value and improved reclassification. Finally, persistently impaired LVGLS in AR is associated with increased mortality.

13. Strain imaging in mixed aortic valve disease

Very little information has been published on the use of strain imaging in the management of patients with mixed aortic valve disease (**Figure 3**). The next paragraph summarizes the findings and conclusions in one study:

- Longitudinal LV function is reduced in both pressure and volume overload, and both of this overload patterns are equally harmful to the ventricle. Gorgulu et al. [49] evaluated a total of 27 subjects with mixed aortic valve disease

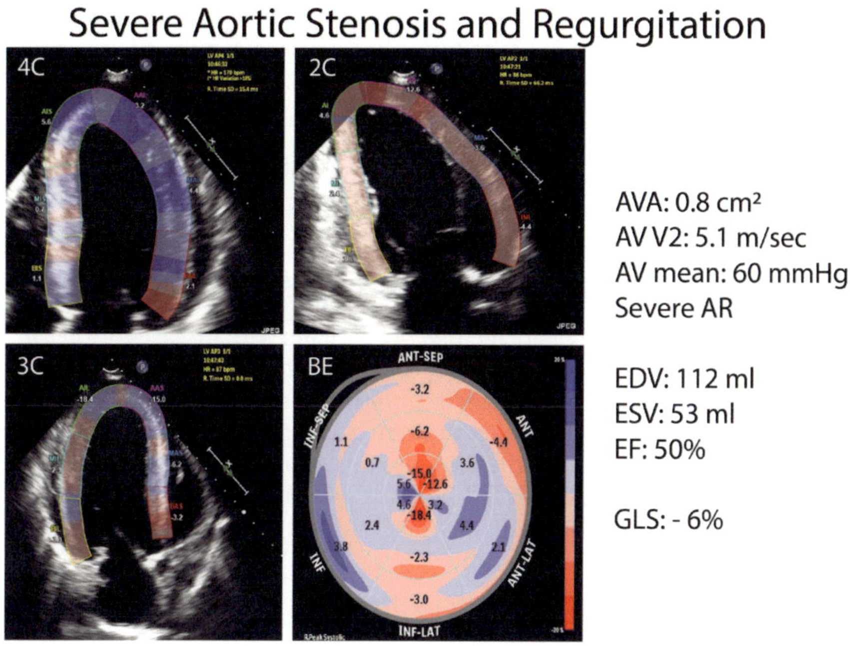

Figure 3.
Severe aortic stenosis and regurgitation: this example illustrates the presence of severe LV dysfunction as demonstrated by a marked drop of GLS to −6% despite a borderline drop of LV ejection fraction to 50%. The combination of severe aortic stenosis and regurgitation likely produces significant volume and pressure overload of the LV with significant LV dysfunction that is unmasked by strain analysis.

(53 ± 15 years). Fifteen healthy subjects (mean age 50 ± 6 years) were enrolled as the control group. Longitudinal peak systolic strain rate values of each segment derived from analysis of a total of 804 segments were significantly decreased in this patient population ($P < 0.001$). Global longitudinal peak systolic strain rate was also significantly decreased in aortic stenosis and regurgitation compared to the control group (−1 ± 0.5, −0.9 ± 0.3, and −1.6 ± 0.3, $P = 0.001$). As far as the comparison between patients with aortic stenosis and aortic regurgitation, neither global strain rate nor strain rate for each myocardial segment was found to be different.

14. Unresolved issues

Although strain analysis is been used with increasing frequency for the evaluation of cardiac function, there are still issues with reproducibility of deformation analysis data, particularly when different echocardiography machines or analysis software is used. Until this issue is resolved the current recommendation is to use the same machine and software when obtaining comparative studies.

The fidelity of the strain data sets is dependent on the quality of the echocardiographic data, unfortunately endocardial contrast enhancing agents cannot be used during strain analysis, therefore strain analysis sometimes has to be obtained with substandard images. The current recommendation is not to report strain values if the echocardiographic images are of poor quality. Hopefully work-around solutions will be found to permit strain analysis with endocardial enhancement agents use.

The current literature supports actionable interventions according to fairly well-defined values of decreased LV ejection fraction, this is not as developed on the characterization of LV dysfunction according to levels of decreased strain values.

Although the literature on strain is fairly robust in aortic stenosis, it is only moderately developed in aortic regurgitation and almost not existent in mixed aortic valve disease.

15. Incorporating strain analysis into clinical practice in aortic valve disease

Despite some of the shortcomings of strain analysis in aortic valve disease we have reviewed, we feel the added value this technique provides, justifies its use in the day to day imaging management of patients with diseases of the aortic valve. Our practice and recommendation is to characterize and sequentially follow global longitudinal strain in patients with moderate and severe aortic stenosis and/or moderate and severe aortic regurgitation. In asymptomatic patients with severe AS or AR and normal EF, the presence of an abnormal GLS should alert the clinician for the need of closer follow up or possibly aortic valve replacement/intervention.

16. Future directions

The following studies highlight areas of study with high potential for development in the area of strain analysis in patients with aortic valve disease.

16.1 Three-dimensional speckle tracking

- Broch et al. [50] studied, 31 patients with moderate to severe AR, 15 elite endurance athletes, and 17 healthy control subjects using three-dimensional speckle-tracking echocardiography. Global circumferential strain (GCS), global longitudinal strain (GLS), end-systolic circumferential wall stress (ESSc), end-systolic meridional wall stress (ESSm), and the wall stress ratio (ESSc/ESSm) were measured. LV end-diastolic volumes were similar in athletes and patients with AR and significantly larger than in healthy control subjects. Values of GLS in control subjects, athletes, and patients with AR were −18.8 ± 1.9%, −17.3 ± 2.0%, and −16.4± 2.0%, respectively (control subjects vs. athletes and patients, $P < .05$), whereas values of GCS were −16.9 ± 2.0%, −15.5 ± 1.9%, and −17.9 ± 2.6%, respectively (athletes vs. control subjects and patients, $P < .01$). The authors concluded that in compensated AR, relatively high GCS compensates for reduced GLS in a manner consistent with the preserved ejection fractions observed in these patients.

16.2 Stress GLS

- Uncovering post-exercise myocardial dysfunction in patients with asymptomatic AS with preserved left ventricular function can aid in risk assessment of these patients [51].

16.3 Multi-layer strain

- Left ventricular myocardial strain gradient using a novel multi-layer transthoracic echocardiography technique positively correlates with severity of aortic stenosis [23].

16.4 Diastolic strain

- Early diastolic strain rate in relation to systolic and diastolic function and prognosis in aortic stenosis [52].

16.5 Left atrial strain

- Preoperative left atrial strain predicts postoperative atrial fibrillation in patients undergoing aortic valve replacement for aortic stenosis [40].

17. Conclusions

Deformation imaging, particularly in the form of global longitudinal strain, has evolved as a powerful tool in the evaluation of ventricular function in patients with aortic valve disease. GLS is particularly suited to detect subclinical LV dysfunction, before a drop in LV ejection fraction, providing the opportunity to intervene earlier to prevent serious and permanent LV dysfunction. The role of GLS in the management of aortic stenosis is quite robust, illuminating nuances of LV dysfunction in aortic valve disease such as impact in severity of AS, prognosis, timing for surgery and interventions, low gradient aortic stenosis and presence of associated coronary artery disease, among others. Similar added value has been demonstrated in the application of GLS in the detection of subclinical LV dysfunction in patients with aortic regurgitation. Very little information exists in the use of GLS in patients with mixed aortic valve disease providing an opportunity for future research in this important group of patients with aortic valve disease.

Author details

Ernesto E. Salcedo[1,2*] and Edward A. Gill[1,2,3]

1 Division of Cardiology, University of Colorado School of Medicine, Anschutz Medical Campus, United States

2 University of Colorado Hospital, Aurora CO, United States

3 Interventional Echocardiography, University of Colorado Hospital, Aurora, CO, United States

*Address all correspondence to: ernesto.e.salcedo@ucdenver.edu

References

[1] Nkomo VT, Gardin JM, Skelton TN, Gottdiener JS, Scott CG, Enriquez-Sarano M. Burden of valvular heart diseases: A population-based study. Lancet. 2006;**368**:1005-1011

[2] Ng ACT, Prihadi EA, Antoni ML, et al. Left ventricular global longitudinal strain is predictive of all-cause mortality independent of aortic stenosis severity and ejection fraction. European Heart Journal Cardiovascular Imaging. 2018;**19**:859-867

[3] Marciniak A, Glover K, Sharma R. Cohort profile: Prevalence of valvular heart disease in community patients with suspected heart failure in UK. BMJ Open. 2017;7:e012240

[4] Ng ACT, Delgado V, Bax JJ. Application of left ventricular strain in patients with aortic and mitral valve disease. Current Opinion in Cardiology. 2018;**33**:470-478

[5] Mor-Avi V, Lang RM, Badano LP, et al. Current and evolving echocardiographic techniques for the quantitative evaluation of cardiac mechanics: ASE/EAE consensus statement on methodology and indications endorsed by the Japanese Society of Echocardiography. Journal of the American Society of Echocardiography. 2011;**24**:277-313

[6] Voigt JU, Pedrizzetti G, Lysyansky P, et al. Definitions for a common standard for 2D speckle tracking echocardiography: Consensus document of the EACVI/ASE/Industry Task Force to standardize deformation imaging. Journal of the American Society of Echocardiography. 2015;**28**:183-193

[7] Nishimura RA, Otto CM, Bonow RO, et al. AHA/ACC focused update of the 2014 AHA/ACC guideline for the management of patients with valvular heart disease: A report of the American College of Cardiology/American Heart Association Task Force on Clinical Practice Guidelines. Journal of the American College of Cardiology. 2017, 2017;**70**:252-289

[8] Baumgartner H, Falk V, Bax JJ, et al. ESC/EACTS guidelines for the management of valvular heart disease. European Heart Journal. 2017, 2017;**38**:2739-2791

[9] Lang RM, Badano LP, Mor-Avi V, et al. Recommendations for cardiac chamber quantification by echocardiography in adults: An update from the American Society of Echocardiography and the European Association of Cardiovascular Imaging. Journal of the American Society of Echocardiography. 2015;**28**:1-39 e14

[10] Vollema EM, Sugimoto T, Shen M, et al. Association of left ventricular global longitudinal strain with asymptomatic severe aortic stenosis: Natural course and prognostic value. JAMA Cardiology. 2018;**3**:839-847

[11] Iwahashi N, Nakatani S, Kanzaki H, Hasegawa T, Abe H, Kitakaze M. Acute improvement in myocardial function assessed by myocardial strain and strain rate after aortic valve replacement for aortic stenosis. Journal of the American Society of Echocardiography. 2006;**19**:1238-1244

[12] Miyazaki S, Daimon M, Miyazaki T, et al. Global longitudinal strain in relation to the severity of aortic stenosis: A two-dimensional speckle-tracking study. Echocardiography. 2011;**28**:703-708

[13] Magne J, Cosyns B, Popescu BA, et al. Distribution and prognostic significance of left ventricular global longitudinal strain in asymptomatic significant aortic stenosis: An individual participant data meta-analysis. JACC: Cardiovascular Imaging. 2019;**12**:84-92

[14] Kearney LG, Lu K, Ord M, et al. Global longitudinal strain is a strong independent predictor of all-cause mortality in patients with aortic stenosis. European Heart Journal Cardiovascular Imaging. 2012;**13**:827-833

[15] Kusunose K, Goodman A, Parikh R, et al. Incremental prognostic value of left ventricular global longitudinal strain in patients with aortic stenosis and preserved ejection fraction. Circulation. Cardiovascular Imaging. 2014;7:938-945

[16] Salaun E, Casalta AC, Donal E, et al. Apical four-chamber longitudinal left ventricular strain in patients with aortic stenosis and preserved left ventricular ejection fraction: Analysis related with flow/gradient pattern and association with outcome. European Heart Journal Cardiovascular Imaging. 2018;**19**:868-878

[17] Fries B, Liu D, Gaudron P, et al. Role of global longitudinal strain in the prediction of outcome in patients with severe aortic valve stenosis. The American Journal of Cardiology. 2017;**120**:640-647

[18] Goodman A, Kusunose K, Popovic ZB, et al. Synergistic utility of brain natriuretic peptide and left ventricular strain in patients with significant aortic stenosis. Journal of the American Heart Association. 2016;**5**:1-11

[19] Kong WKF, Vollema EM, Prevedello F, et al. Prognostic implications of left ventricular global longitudinal strain in patients with bicuspid aortic valve disease and preserved left ventricular ejection fraction. European Heart Journal Cardiovascular Imaging. 2019;**21**:759-767

[20] Carstensen HG, Larsen LH, Hassager C, Kofoed KF, Jensen JS, Mogelvang R. Association of ischemic heart disease to global and regional longitudinal strain in asymptomatic aortic stenosis. The International Journal of Cardiovascular Imaging. 2015;**31**:485-495

[21] Ilardi F, Marchetta S, Martinez C, et al. Impact of aortic stenosis on layer-specific longitudinal strain: Relationship with symptoms and outcome. European Heart Journal Cardiovascular Imaging. 2019;**21**:408-416

[22] Hyodo E, Arai K, Koczo A, et al. Alteration in subendocardial and subepicardial myocardial strain in patients with aortic valve stenosis: An early marker of left ventricular dysfunction? Journal of the American Society of Echocardiography. 2012;**25**:153-159

[23] Fung MJ, Thomas L, Leung DY. Alterations in layer-specific left ventricular global longitudinal and circumferential strain in patients with aortic stenosis: A comparison of aortic valve replacement versus conservative management over a 12-month period. Journal of the American Society of Echocardiography. 2019;**32**:92-101

[24] Fung MJ, Leung DY, Thomas L. Differential myocardial fibre involvement by strain analysis in patients with aortic stenosis. Heart, Lung & Circulation. 2018;**27**:1357-1367

[25] Delgado V, Tops LF, van Bommel RJ, et al. Strain analysis in patients with severe aortic stenosis and preserved left ventricular ejection fraction undergoing surgical valve replacement. European Heart Journal. 2009;**30**:3037-3047

[26] Lee SP, Kim YJ, Kim JH, et al. Deterioration of myocardial function in paradoxical low-flow severe aortic stenosis: Two-dimensional strain analysis. Journal of the American Society of Echocardiography. 2011;**24**:976-983

[27] Bartko PE, Heinze G, Graf S, et al. Two-dimensional strain for the assessment of left ventricular function in low flow-low gradient aortic stenosis, relationship to hemodynamics, and outcome: A substudy of the multicenter TOPAS study. Circulation. Cardiovascular Imaging. 2013;**6**:268-276

[28] Sato K, Seo Y, Ishizu T, et al. Prognostic value of global longitudinal strain in paradoxical low-flow, low-gradient severe aortic stenosis with preserved ejection fraction. Circulation Journal. 2014;**78**:2750-2759

[29] Holmes AA, Taub CC, Garcia MJ, Shan J, Slovut DP. Paradoxical low-flow aortic stenosis is defined by increased ventricular hydraulic load and reduced longitudinal strain. Journal of Cardiovascular Medicine (Hagerstown, Md.). 2017;**18**:87-95

[30] Dahou A, Bartko PE, Capoulade R, et al. Usefulness of global left ventricular longitudinal strain for risk stratification in low ejection fraction, low-gradient aortic stenosis: Results from the multicenter true or pseudo-severe aortic stenosis study. Circulation. Cardiovascular Imaging. 2015;**8**:e002117

[31] Dahou A, Clavel MA, Capoulade R, et al. Right ventricular longitudinal strain for risk stratification in low-flow, low-gradient aortic stenosis with low ejection fraction. Heart. 2016;**102**:548-554

[32] Tadic M, Cuspidi C, Pencic B, et al. The impact of arterial hypertension on left ventricular strain in patients with aortic stenosis and preserved ejection fraction. Journal of Hypertension. 2018;**37**:747-753

[33] Cramariuc D, Gerdts E, Hjertaas JJ, Cramariuc A, Davidsen ES, Matre K. Myocardial function in aortic stenosis—Insights from radial multilayer Doppler strain. Cardiovascular Ultrasound. 2015;**13**:8

[34] Poulsen SH, Sogaard P, Nielsen-Kudsk JE, Egeblad H. Recovery of left ventricular systolic longitudinal strain after valve replacement in aortic stenosis and relation to natriuretic peptides. Journal of the American Society of Echocardiography. 2007;**20**:877-884

[35] Dahl JS, Videbaek L, Poulsen MK, Rudbaek TR, Pellikka PA, Moller JE. Global strain in severe aortic valve stenosis: Relation to clinical outcome after aortic valve replacement. Circulation. Cardiovascular Imaging. 2012;**5**:613-620

[36] Marcus KA, de Korte CL, Feuth T, et al. Persistent reduction in left ventricular strain using two-dimensional speckle-tracking echocardiography after balloon valvuloplasty in children with congenital valvular aortic stenosis. Journal of the American Society of Echocardiography. 2012;**25**:473-485

[37] Kafa R, Kusunose K, Goodman AL, et al. Association of abnormal postoperative left ventricular global longitudinal strain with outcomes in severe aortic stenosis following aortic valve replacement. JAMA Cardiology. 2016;**1**:494-496

[38] Naji P, Shah S, Svensson LG, et al. Incremental prognostic use of left ventricular global longitudinal strain in asymptomatic/minimally symptomatic patients with severe bioprosthetic aortic stenosis undergoing redo aortic valve replacement. Circulation. Cardiovascular Imaging. 2017;**10**:1-10

[39] Lisi M, Henein MY, Cameli M, et al. Severity of aortic stenosis predicts early post-operative normalization of left atrial size and function detected by myocardial strain. International Journal of Cardiology. 2013;**167**:1450-1455

[40] Cameli M, Lisi M, Reccia R, et al. Pre-operative left atrial strain predicts post-operative atrial fibrillation in patients undergoing aortic valve

replacement for aortic stenosis. The International Journal of Cardiovascular Imaging. 2014;**30**:279-286

[41] Gelsomino S, Luca F, Parise O, et al. Longitudinal strain predicts left ventricular mass regression after aortic valve replacement for severe aortic stenosis and preserved left ventricular function. Heart and Vessels. 2013;**28**:775-784

[42] Marciniak A, Sutherland GR, Marciniak M, Claus P, Bijnens B, Jahangiri M. Myocardial deformation abnormalities in patients with aortic regurgitation: A strain rate imaging study. European Journal of Echocardiography. 2009;**10**:112-119

[43] Smedsrud MK, Pettersen E, Gjesdal O, et al. Detection of left ventricular dysfunction by global longitudinal systolic strain in patients with chronic aortic regurgitation. Journal of the American Society of Echocardiography. 2011;**24**:1253-1259

[44] Di Salvo G, Rea A, Mormile A, et al. Usefulness of bidimensional strain imaging for predicting outcome in asymptomatic patients aged </= 16 years with isolated moderate to severe aortic regurgitation. The American Journal of Cardiology. 2012;**110**:1051-1055

[45] Kaneko A, Tanaka H, Onishi T, et al. Subendocardial dysfunction in patients with chronic severe aortic regurgitation and preserved ejection fraction detected with speckle-tracking strain imaging and transmural myocardial strain profile. European Heart Journal Cardiovascular Imaging. 2013;**14**:339-346

[46] Park SH, Yang YA, Kim KY, et al. Left ventricular strain as predictor of chronic aortic regurgitation. Journal of Cardiovascular Ultrasound. 2015;**23**:78-85

[47] Alashi A, Mentias A, Abdallah A, et al. Incremental prognostic utility of left ventricular global longitudinal strain in asymptomatic patients with significant chronic aortic regurgitation and preserved left ventricular ejection fraction. JACC: Cardiovascular Imaging. 2018;**11**:673-682

[48] Alashi A, Khullar T, Mentias A, et al. Long-term outcomes after aortic valve surgery in patients with asymptomatic chronic aortic regurgitation and preserved LVEF: Impact of baseline and follow-up global longitudinal strain. JACC: Cardiovascular Imaging. 2020;**13**:12-21

[49] Gorgulu S, Norgaz T, Nurkalem Z, et al. Comparison of left ventricular contractility in pressure and volume overload: A strain rate study in the clinical model of aortic stenosis and regurgitation. Echocardiography. 2010;**27**:798-802

[50] Broch K, de Marchi SF, Massey R, et al. Left ventricular contraction pattern in chronic aortic regurgitation and preserved ejection fraction: Simultaneous stress-strain analysis by three-dimensional echocardiography. Journal of the American Society of Echocardiography. 2017;**30**:422-430 e2

[51] Levy-Neuman S, Meledin V, Gandelman G, et al. The association between longitudinal strain at rest and stress and outcome in asymptomatic patients with moderate and severe aortic stenosis. Journal of the American Society of Echocardiography. 2019;**32**:722-729

[52] Dahl JS, Barros-Gomes S, Videbaek L, et al. Early diastolic strain rate in relation to systolic and diastolic function and prognosis in aortic stenosis. JACC: Cardiovascular Imaging. 2016;**9**:519-528

Chapter 4

Current and Future Management Strategies of Type A Aortic Dissection

Imran Khan, Prashant Joshi, Adrian W. Pick and Julian A. Smith

Abstract

Type A Aortic dissection is a life-threatening emergency. It has varied clinical presentation from acute severe chest pain radiating to the back, collapse due to aortic rupture or pericardial tamponade or features of myocardial infarction, end organ or limb ischemia. The outcome is determined by the extent of the dissection, timing of presentation, comorbid factors, prompt diagnosis, adequate cerebral protection strategies, and skilled post-operative intensive care. Good immediate and mid-term results have been obtained with standard surgical techniques of aortic root, ascending aorta +/− hemi arch replacement. Endovascular techniques can be used as a hybrid procedure to provide more durable long term results.

Keywords: dissection, cerebral protection strategies, aortic root, ascending aorta, hemi arch, endovascular techniques

1. Introduction

Type A aortic dissection is a life threatening condition requiring emergency surgical intervention. Statistics show an incidence of approximately three cases per 100,000 per year [1, 2]. Data analysis from the International Registry of Acute Aortic Dissections (IRAD) reported a predominant male patient population and a mean age of 63 years at presentation [3]. Surgical repair for Type A Aortic dissection is challenging, the complexity proportionate to the location and extent of aortic tissue dissected, cardiac complications and end organ ischemia. The current standard surgical approach includes replacement of the aortic root (Bentall technique) or valve sparing root replacement, isolated ascending aorta replacement, and hemi or full arch replacement. Recent advances include frozen elephant trunk (FET) technique, total aortic repair, endovascular and hybrid approaches and stenting. All of these surgical approaches, including classification, clinical presentation, risk factors, diagnosis, pre-operative preparation, cannulation strategies, and cerebral protection will be discussed in this review.

2. Classification

The Stanford classification (1970) is the most commonly used system (**Figure 1**) [4]. It does not classify the site of tear. It is more of a clinically useful classification

IntechOpen

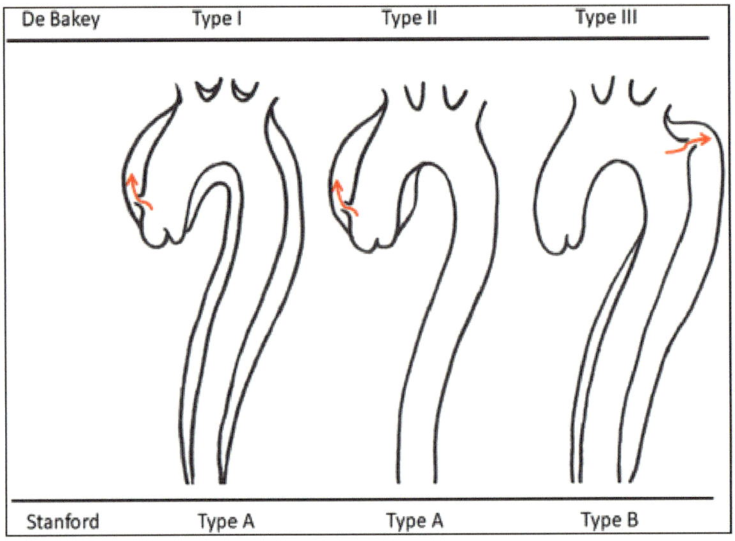

Figure 1.
Stanford and DeBakey classification.

to guide acute management. Stanford type A involves ascending aorta proximal to innominate artery, irrespective of involvement of aortic arch or descending aorta. Stanford type B dissection involves only the thoracic aorta distal to the left subclavian artery [5]. Intimal tears originating distal to left subclavian artery but dissecting retrogradely into ascending aorta will be type A. Intimal tears starting in the aortic arch and extending into ascending aorta are type A and extending into descending aorta are type B. If the intimal tear is restricted to aortic arch, then it is type non-A non-B.

The DeBakey type I involves ascending aorta and extends beyond the innominate artery. Type II involves only the ascending aorta. Type III involves thoracic aorta distal to left subclavian artery. It is more useful for long-term follow-up as it differentiates between proximal and distal aortic dissection extent (**Figure 1**) [4].

The Penn classification is a recently introduced method of classifying based on clinical presentation [6]. Class Aa—absence of branch vessel malperfusion or circulatory collapse; Class Ab—symptoms or signs of localised organ ischemia; Class Ac—circulatory collapse with or without cardiac involvement; Class Abc—combined localised and generalised ischemia.

3. Risk factors

Men form approximately 62–68% of all patients undergoing surgery [7]. The triad of hypertension (67–86% patients), smoking and atherosclerosis is an independent predictor of type A aortic dissection [8]. Data correlating the risk of aortic dissection in bicuspid aortic valve is limited and controversial. However, some centres advocate early prophylactic ascending aortic replacement in patients with aortas larger than approximately 5.0 cm in diameter or with a cross-sectional area to height ratio greater than approximately 10 cm^2/m [9]. In the NORCAAD registry, 6% patients were reported to have bicuspid aortic valve [7]. The Marfan syndrome is present in around 4% of ATAAD patients in NORCAAD registry [10]. The patients typically have pear-shaped aneurysm of aortic root. Due to mutation in FBN1 gene, there is decreased strength and elasticity of elastin—rich tissue of aortic wall. Predominantly, medium and large sized arteries are involved in dissection (**Table 1**).

(1) Cardiovascular and life style factors
Uncontrolled hypertension
Age
Smoking
Dyslipidemia
Cocaine
Pregnancy
(2) Congenital and connective tissue
Bicuspid aortic valve
Marfan syndrome
(3) Iatrogenic
Coronary catheterisation
Arterial cannulation
Aortic cross clamping
IABP
(4) Vascular inflammation
Takayasu arteritis
(5) Trauma
Deceleration injury

Table 1.
Risk factors for acute aortic dissection.

4. Clinical presentation

TAAD patients (85%) typically present with sudden intense central chest pain (ripping or tearing) radiating to the neck, back or abdomen. [11]. ECG abnormalities (50% patients) include ST/T wave changes, conduction defects, and arrhythmias. This sometimes leads to the misdiagnosis of myocardial infarction leading to fatal mistake of giving antiplatelet therapy or thrombolysis. This delays the diagnosis and increases peri-operative bleeding complications. Aortic regurgitation (70% patients) can occur through prolapse of right or non- coronary valve cusps and detachment of commissures. Pulmonary oedema may occur through acute dilation of the left ventricle. Haemorrhagic pericardial tamponade is a very strong predictor of aortic dissection. Reduced or absent femoral pulses are seen. Neurological sequlae include syncope, stroke. Mal-perfusion of spinal cord leads to paraplegia. Acute renal failure and mesenteric ischemia are seen if the dissection involves descending thoracic and abdominal aorta [12]. Rupture of the aneurysm is immediately fatal.

5. Diagnosis

1. **Clinical**: Constellation of findings of chest pain, diastolic murmur, blood pressure difference in both upper limbs, pulse deficit, neurological sequelae are good indicators for TAAD [13].

2. **Chest X ray** (**Figure 2**) shows widened mediastinum (49% patients), which is non-specific [14].

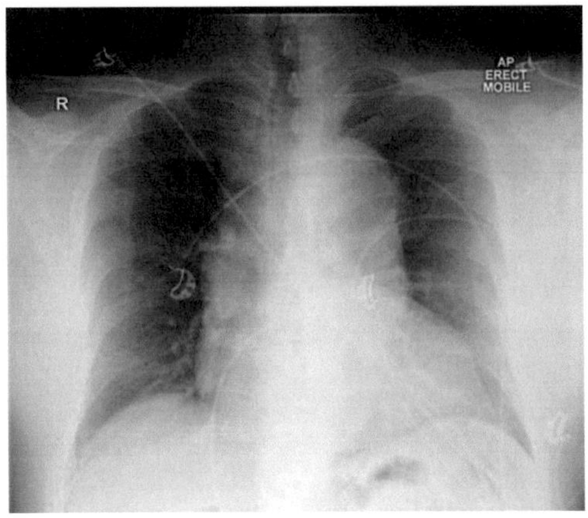

Figure 2.
Chest X-ray of a patient with ATAD showing a widened mediastinum.

3. **ECG** may show ST-T changes especially in right coronary territory, non-specific changes of left ventricle hypertrophy, pericardial effusion

4. **CT scan** (**Figure 3**): the most reliable diagnostic tool for acute aortic dissection. It is available in almost every hospital and can be rapidly performed. Sensitivity and specificity is excellent [15]

The following information may be provided from a CT-scan:

a. Detection of the true and false lumen in the dissected aorta

b. Identification of the site of the intimal tear The extent of the dissection

c. Arch vessel and thoracic and abdominal branch vessel involvement

d. Planning the site of cannulation

Limitations of CT-scanning include not providing information about dissection entry site and functional status of the heart.

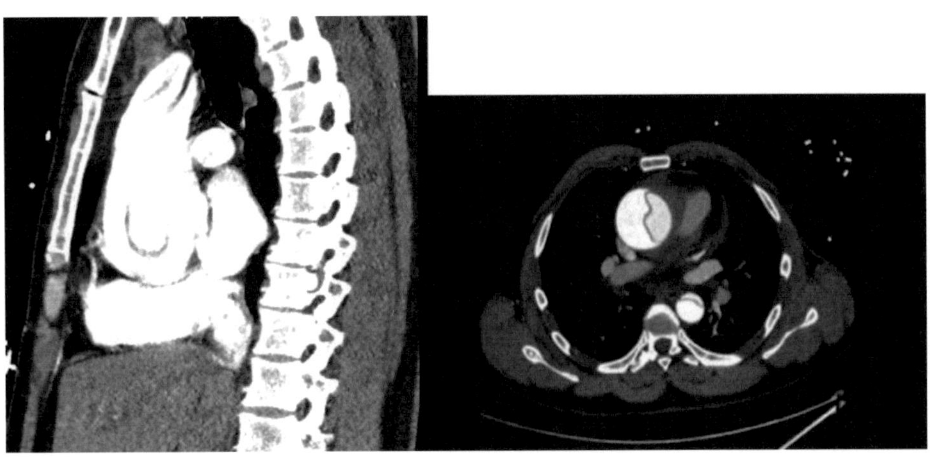

Figure 3.
CT-scan of a patient with TAAD.

5. Trans-oesophageal echocardiography (TEE; **Figure 4**)

TEE is portable, less invasive and has sensitivity and specificity approximately 100% [16]. It provides information about:

a. The dissection flap and false lumen in ascending aorta

b. The entry site of tear using colour Doppler

c. Coronary ostial obstruction due to the dissection

d. Dilation of aorta and left ventricle function

e. Pericardial effusion and tamponade

f. Aortic regurgitation and anatomy of aortic root

g. Has a better window than TTE to visualise aortic arch and descending aorta

h. Pleural effusion

Limitations include difficulty in visualisation of the proximal arch due to the interposition of bronchial air [17].

6. **Magnetic resonance imaging (MRI)**

MRI is an accurate investigative modality for acute aortic dissection (sensitivity and specificity, 98%) [18]. It is rarely used in the setting of TAAD where most of the patients are wheeled into operating room as soon as the diagnosis is made. It may have a small role in those patients allergic to iodinated contrast agents or in patients with acute renal failure who are stable enough to undergo MRI.

7. **Preoperative coronary angiography:**

Its role is controversial [19]. Justification of not performing cardiac catheterisation include risk of catheter induced aortic rupture and delaying surgery where percentage mortality increases by 1 % every hour [20].

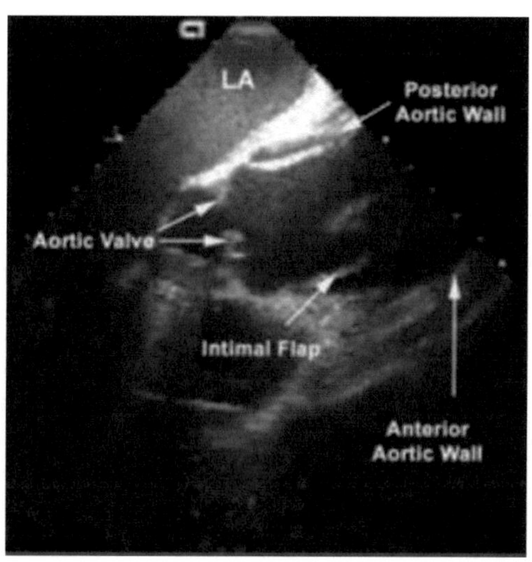

Figure 4.
TEE of a patient with ATAD.

6. Surgical strategies

6.1 Preparation for surgery

1. Blood pressure (BP) control: One of the most important pre-requisites of successful outcome is very strict control of BP. Systolic BP should be less than 110 mmHg. It can be lowered using intravenous beta blocker (esmolol) or combined alpha & beta receptor antagonists (labetalol) or glyceryl trinitrate. Intravenous adrenaline should be used in patients presenting with cardiogenic shock and cardiac tamponade. Anaesthetic induction is also another step where BP should be tightly controlled. Commonly used medications include Fentanyl, isoflurane and glyceryl trinitrate. Peri-operatively, a target systolic blood pressure of 90–110 mmHg, mean arterial pressure of 60 mmHg, and central venous pressure of 8–12 mmHg are recommended [21].

2. Coagulation status: Aortic dissection activates inflammatory, coagulation and fibrinolytic pathways leading to disseminated intravascular coagulation. Consumption coagulopathy is worsened in some patients by inadvertently prescribing aspirin, clopidogrel by misdiagnosing these patients as having acute coronary syndromes. Hence, adequate amounts of packed red blood cells, platelets, fresh frozen plasma and cryoprecipiate should be kept ready for use.

3. 2 arterial lines (both arms) should be placed to monitor differential blood pressures.

Also include a femoral arterial line to monitor distal perfusion pressures

4. Cerebral oxygenation monitoring by near—infrared spectroscopy

5. Invasive monitoring of intracranial pressure by lumbar catheter (occasionally)

7. Cannulation strategies

1. Femoral artery cannulation (**Figure 5**)

For many years, it has been the cannulation site of choice [22]. Allowing rapid access, it is usually used in hemodynamically unstable patients, especially with impending cardiac tamponade and aortic rupture. It is important to mark the femoral artery before skin preparation as it may be difficult to localise it during hypotension. Common femoral artery is situated medial and inferior to the midpoint of the inguinal ligament. An oblique or vertical incision may be used for exposure [23]. An open Seldinger technique is quick and can be performed with minimal dissection. Advantages of this approach include (i) cardiopulmonary bypass is established quickly, (ii) easy to access with a closed chest, (iii) less likely to be dissected, (iv) prevents aortic rupture in patients with cardiac tamponade. Disadvantages include (i) stroke and malperfusion due to dynamic obstruction and (ii) retrograde perfusion leading to embolic complications due to atherosclerotic emboli. The femoral artery with a dissection flap is not used for cannulation.

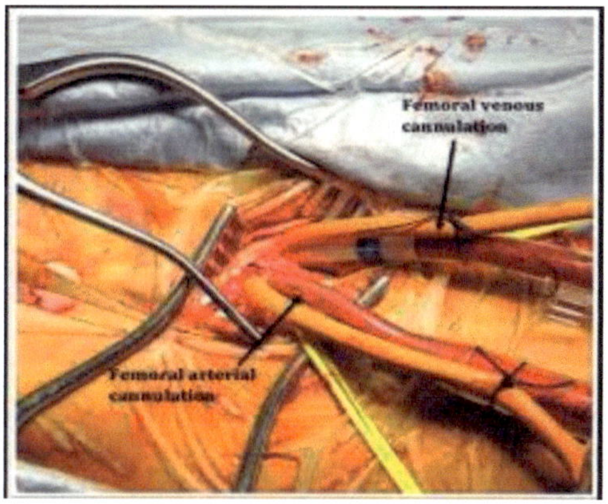

Figure 5.
Femoral artery cannulation.

2. Axillary artery cannulation (**Figure 6**)

Introduced in 1990s [24], axillary artery cannulation is gaining greater acceptance among surgeons as they switch to an antegrade perfusion strategy. It is more commonly used in hemodynamically stable patients. Infraclavicular dissection exposes the first part of axillary artery [25]. The pectoralis major muscle is split. The neurovascular bundle is situated deep in the clavipectoral fascia. The deltopectoral approach exposes the second and third parts for cannulation [26]. The axillary artery can be directly cannulated or anastomosed with end to side 8 mm vascular graft. Advantages include (i) antegrade perfusion flow and (ii) can be used for antegrade cerebral perfusion by occluding innominate artery. Disadvantages of this approach include (i) takes more time than femoral cannulation especially in obese patients and (ii) technically more difficult and risk of injury to brachial plexus nerves.

3. Central aortic cannulation:

Locating a site where the chances of not entering into the false lumen is the most critical part. It can be done with TEE, CT or epiaortic scanning. Cannulation can be performed with Seldinger technique or directly. Advantages include (i) CPB

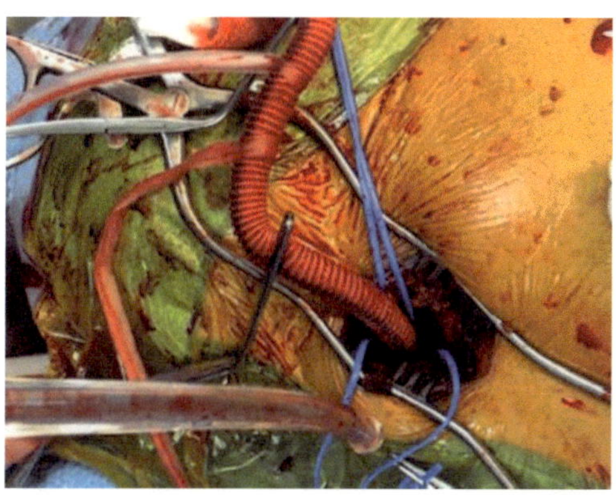

Figure 6.
Axillary artery cannulation.

established quickly in unstable patients and (ii) antegrade flow. Disadvantages include (i) rupture of cannulation site and (ii) false lumen perfusion [27].

8. Peri-aortic dissection before Going on CPB and after cardiac arrest

1. An expeditious midline sternotomy should be done with SBP maintained around 100–110 mmHg. The dissected aorta is usually dilated, thinned out and blood seeping through adventitial layers (**Figure 7**).

2. Upon opening the pericardium, be prepared for free aortic rupture (**Figure 8**). To minimise the risk either (i) femoral arterial and venous cannula should be in place or (ii) if axillary artery cannulation is done, then the surgeon should be prepared to quickly place the two-stage cannula into right atrium.

3. Patient is cooled to a core temperature of 26–28°C. For hemi-arch replacement and short duration of total hypothermic circulatory arrest, 27°C temperature is optimum. If total arch replacement is planned, then the patient can be further cooled to 22–24°C.

4. After going on CPB, a left ventricular vent is placed to prevent left ventricular distension due to associated acute aortic regurgitation. Retrogarde cardioplegia catheter is placed to arrest the heart, as antegrade cardioplegic arrest may not be possible due to aortic regurgitation. After the cardiac arrest and upon opening the aorta, antegrade ostial cardioplegia can be administered.

5. If the patient is stable, innominate artery is carefully dissected and looped with a vascular loop before going on CPB. This can be occluded or clamped later to provide antegrade cerebral perfusion through the previously cannulated axillary artery.

6. After going on CPB, the aorta is dissected free from surrounding adhesions. When creating the plane between ascending aorta and main pulmonary artery, it is important to retain as much adventitial tissue on the aortic side.

7. It is important to identify right pulmonary artery and avoid injuring it, while dissecting ascending aorta.

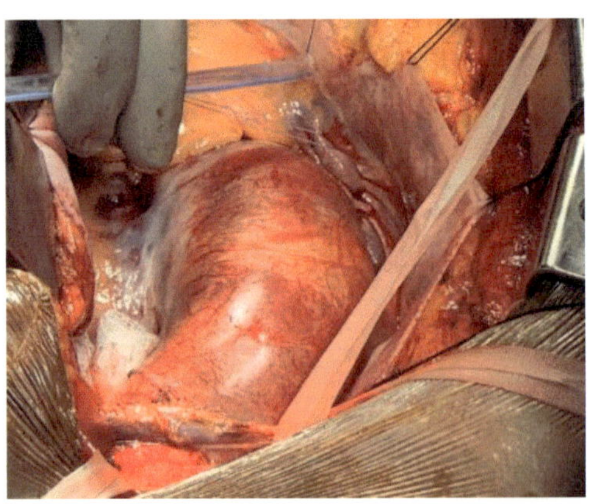

Figure 7.
The dissected ascending aorta.

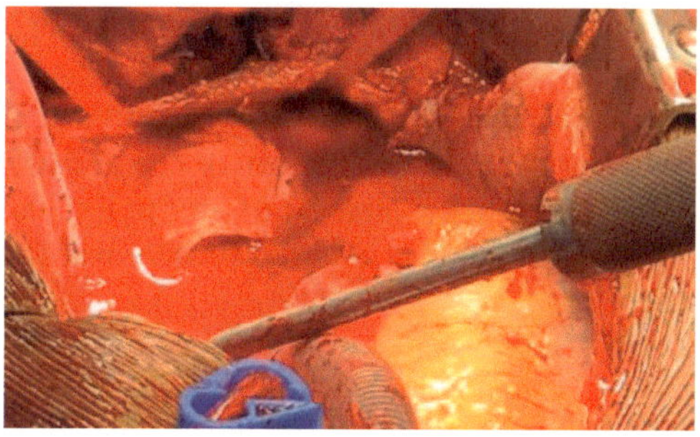

Figure 8.
Aortic rupture prior to establishing CPB.

8. Clamp the aorta somewhere in the mid-ascending aorta, which will be eventually resected while doing open distal anastomoses. This allows assessment of the site of the tear and of the aortic root and also minimises the total circulatory arrest time.

9. While excising the dissected ascending aorta, it is important to avoid injury to the main and right pulmonary artery.

10. While dissecting towards aortic root, left and right coronary ostia are identified and coronary buttons prepared (if aortic root replacement is planned).

9. Hypothermic circulatory cardiac arrest and cerebral protection strategies

Because of the low threshold tolerance to ischemia, brain protection is of paramount importance during aortic arch procedures. Hypothermia is an option to increase the ischemic time. However, there are limitations of hypothermia and hypothermic circulatory arrest. Protective effects of hypothermia last no more than 9 minutes at 30°, 14 minutes at 25°, 21 minutes at 2°, 31 minutes at 15° and 45 minutes at 10° [28]. Neurological deficits are seen in elderly patients subjected to hypothermic circulatory arrest exceeding 25 minutes.

Several cerebral perfusion techniques have been introduced to extend the safe period of arch repair without residual neurological deficits. Retrograde cerebral perfusion (RCP) in tandem with hypothermic circulatory arrest was introduced in 1990 by Ueda et al. [29] Because the cerebral venous sinuses have no valves, RCP was proposed to provide retrograde perfusion and cooling of central nervous system (CNS). It offered to back-flush air emboli and debris from the cerebral circulation. Neuroprotective effects were most likely related to cooling rather than true nutritive flow [30]. It was also found to provide limited benefit in patients with significant carotid stenosis and vascular anomalies (e.g. an incomplete Circle of Willis) [31].

Antegrade selective cerebral perfusion (SCP) was introduced by Jean Bachet and Daniel Guilmet in Europe [32] and by Teruhisa Kazui in Japan in 1986 [33]. This new perfusion method of "cold cerebroplegia" in combination with hypothermia significantly reduced neurologic complications. Antegrade selective perfusion can be established either by direct cannulation or by anastomosing a prosthetic graft. The options for locating such are (i) right subclavian artery, (ii) innominate artery, (iii) right common carotid artery. These may be combined with left common carotid artery cannulation to provide bilateral antegrade cerebral perfusion.

Direct cannulation is limited by high risk of embolism due to plaque mobilisation from manipulation or by jet flow [34].

Axillary artery cannulation can be used to provide unilateral antegrade SCP during hypothermic arrest without manipulation of the arch vessels. This can be combined with balloon occludable perfusion catheter to left carotid artery to provide bilateral antegrade SCP. To avoid steal, an occlusive balloon catheter is inserted in left subclavian artery.

Unilateral antegrade SCP is sufficient for majority of patients with no pathology of the arch vessels and cerebral vessels. Adequate backflow from the contralateral carotid artery suggests good collateralisation. Near-infrared spectroscopy (NIRS) monitoring can also help to exclude contralateral malperfusion. Bilateral cerebral perfusion may be useful in patients with carotid artery stenosis, previous stroke or cerebrovascular anomalies (incomplete Circle of Willis). Malvindi concluded in his review that "While both unilateral and bilateral ASCP are acceptable, bilateral antegrade cerebral perfusion is safer, when the antegrade SCP time is more than 40-50 minute" [35].

Cerebral perfusion is performed at a rate of 8–12 cc/min/kg body weight, perfusion pressure of 40–60 mmHg at 23–28°C. Alpha stat pH management compared to pH stat management prevents "luxury perfusion" by marinating cerebral autoregulation decreasing the risk of embolization [35].

10. Technical aspects of surgical repair

10.1 Aortic root management

The aortic root is frequently involved with aortic valve rendered incompetent due to commissural dehiscence or annular dilation. Grade II and grade III aortic regurgitation was found in 40 and 23% patients, respectively, in German Registry for Acute Aortic Dissection type A (GERAADA) [36]. There are different surgical approaches for management of aortic root replacement—an aggressive or a more conservative approach.

According to the International Registry of Acute Dissection (IRAD), aortic root replacement compared with conservative root management is not associated with increased in-hospital mortality. In 1995 patients, 18 and 21.3% hospital mortality was found in root replacement and conservative root group respectively (OR 0.989; CI 0.710–1.379; $p = 0.949$). Mid-term results at 3 years showed a survival of 91.6+/1.3% and 92.5+/1.7% for conservative root management and root replacement group, respectively [37].

Indications to perform root replacement in a patient with ATAD include:

1. younger age
2. Marfan syndrome
3. bicuspid aortic valve
4. known aortic valve disease
5. moderate or severe aortic valve insufficiency
6. previous aortic valve replacement
7. large diameter aortic annulus, sinuses of Valsalva and ascending aorta

8. coronary artery involvement

9. aortic root as the most proximal site of dissection

Proximal reconstruction technical (**Figures 9** and **10**) details: After the excision of the dissected aortic root, aortic root reconstruction is done.

Technical principles include:

i. Obliteration of false lumen.

ii. To take the maximum possible adventitia in the anastomoses.

iii. Needle should enter the tissue at right angle to avoid tearing of needle holes.

iv. Sutures should be spaced uniformly and pulled just enough tight to prevent cutting through the fragile tissue.

v. To avoid distortion of the aortic valve, the planar relationship between the graft and sinotubular junction should be maintained.

The Bentall procedure [38] is a fairly standard procedure. It includes anastomosing the composite graft to the aortic annulus and reimplantation of coronary arteries. Patients with type A aortic dissection usually have normal aortic valve cusps, as the pathology is usually limited to the aortic wall.

Valve sparing root replacement is a viable option in hemodynamically stable young patients. But it is technically more complex than straight aortic root replacement. It involves replacing the aortic root by composite graft without replacing the aortic valve. The native aortic root must be dissected from surrounding structures to 2 mm below the nadir of the aortic annulus. Coronary ostia are reimplanted into the graft. It is used to treat aortic regurgitation due to annular enlargement. Contraindications include significant cardiomyopathy, malperfusion, coronary artery disease, >65 years age.

Results from Emory in a 43 patients showed operative mortality of 4.7%. Freedom from aortic valve replacement was 100% and freedom from more than mild aortic regurgitation was 94% at 9 years follow-up. No aortic root reinterventions were required in this series [39].

Conservative approaches to the aortic root (CRR)—In most of the patients presenting with TAAD, the most common pathology seen is a primary intimal tear in the ascending aorta with dissection flap extending to non-coronary cusp. Left and right coronary sinuses are relatively preserved. Any aortic regurgitation

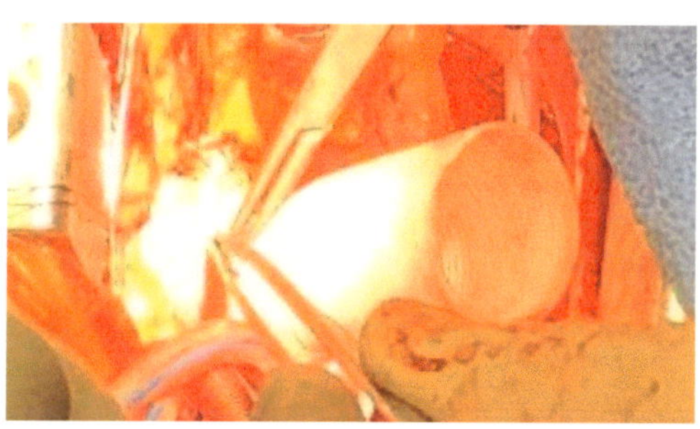

Figure 9.
Aortic root replacement (right coronary ostial anastomosis).

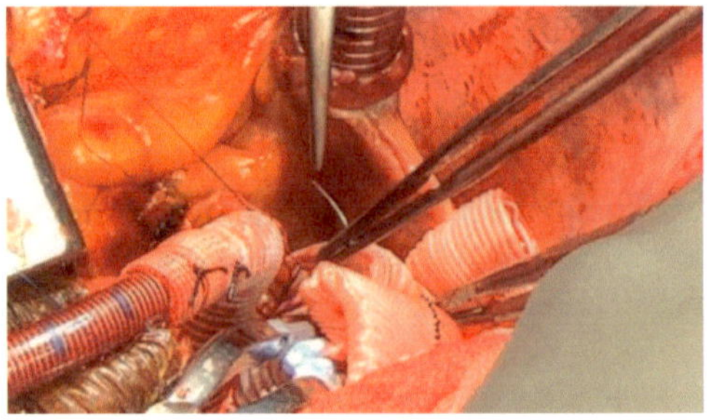

Figure 10.
Proximal anastomoses of aortic root.

is due to unhinging of one of the aortic valve commissural posts. The dissected sinus segments are preserved and supported with resuspension of the native valve commissural posts or prosthetic ascending aorta replacement. The advantages are that it preserves the native sinus tissue, coronary ostia are not reimplanted, shorter ischemic time, avoiding life-long anticoagulation [40]. The most commonly used methods to fortify the aortic wall include Teflon felt and biologic glue. University of Pennsylvania in their series of 489 patients showed freedom from reoperation with this technique of 96, 92 and 89% at 1, 10 and 15 years respectively. The operative mortality was 11% [41].

11. Ascending aorta

The entry site of the dissection tear is usually found the ascending aorta, which is at very high risk of rupture. After excising the dissected portion of ascending aorta, supracommissural ascending aorta replacement can be performed. Open distal anastomoses can be done under hypothermic circulatory arrest after releasing the cross clamp. This facilitates inspection of the aortic arch and if required, arch repair can be undertaken. Also, it is technically much easier to construct a very distal ascending aortic anastomoses. Around 5.6% patients underwent ascending aorta replacement in GERAADA survey [42]. But this procedure also allows for subsequent aneurysmal dilation of the remaining portion of the aorta [43].

12. Hemi-arch or full arch

When the aortic arch is examined during hypothermic circulatory arrest to look for intimal or re-entry tears, a decision is made whether an aortic arch replacement has to be done. The pre-operative CT aortogram helps in localising the dissection and also on deciding the placement of the aortic cross clamp. If the tear is in the ascending aorta or start of the aortic curvature, then hemi-arch replacement is required. If the dissection is extends more distally, a total aortic arch repair should be performed (**Figure 11a**, **b**).

Indications for arch replacement include:

1. Pre-existing aneurysm of the arch

2. Primary intimal tear in distal arch or descending thoracic aorta

3. Secondary intimal tear in arch >10 mm

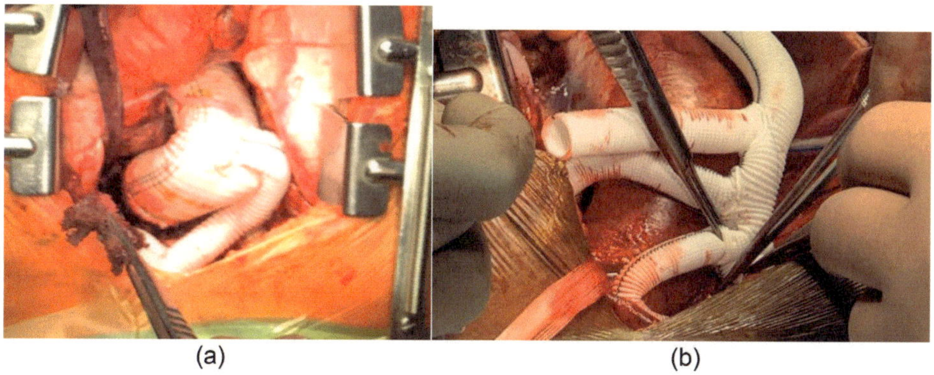

Figure 11.
Total arch replacement. (a, b) Debranching of aortic arch vessels – innominate , carotid artery and left subclavian artery.

4. False lumen more than 22 mm

5. Descending thoracic aorta diameter more than 35 mm

A study of 188 patients by Kim et al. [44] showed that 5 year survival was lower in patients with total arch replacement compared to patients who had hemi-arch repair (65.8% vs. 83.2%, p = 0.013). Neurological complications were higher in total arch repair group compared to hemi-arch (56.9% vs. 24.8%, p < 0.001).There was a direct correlation between patent false lumen in aortic arch or descending aorta and re-intervention. The German registry for TAAD showed no significant difference in peri-operative outcomes between both groups [45]. This group suggested a more aggressive approach to reduce the rate of interventions.

13. Frozen elephant trunk (FET)

The immediate post-operative results have improved post type A Aortic dissection repair. However, long-term results are guarded by the need for aortic re-interventions due to residual dissection and patent false lumen extending into descending thoracic aorta [46]. The frozen elephant trunk technique involves total arch replacement and per-procedural deployment of stent through the true aortic lumen. It is more complex and takes more time. However, there is 90% chance of false lumen obliteration and reduced rates of re-intervention and improved long-term survival [47]. Uchida et al. [47] showed improved survival in the FET group at 5 years (95.3% vs. 69%, p = 0.03) and 100% thrombosis of false lumen in FET group compared to 29% patent false lumen in the non-FET group. However, both groups had similar operative mortality. Caution should be exercised that it should be done in high volume centres and by experienced suregons.as the total duration of hypothermic circulatory arrest can be dramatically increased.

14. Total aortic repair

Deployment of stent in the descending thoracic aorta has its drawbacks. Stent induced false lumen thrombosis activated inflammatory markers like metalloproteinases and proinflammatory cytokines [48], which contribute in the progression of aneurysm by destruction of the extracellular matrix in the aortic wall and neo-angiogenesis. Risk factors for the late development of aneurysm include (i) patent false lumen, (ii) helicoidal flow distal to the endoprosthesis, (iii) aortic wall shear stress gets modified.

Matalanis [49] has introduced the concept of total aortic repair to prevent the above mentioned complication. Patients presenting with TAAD and a descending thoracic aorta diameter of more than 40 mm can benefited from this approach. The repair involves a "Branch first "total aortic arch repair and surgical ascending aorta repair. Second part included endovascular treatment of descending aorta. It includes covered stent graft deployment in the proximal part of descending aorta and rupture of the intimal flap for the last part of aorta. The rupture is managed with the deployment and dilation under balloon of uncovered stent graft. With this approach, aneurysmal dilatation of the false channel is avoided by the creation of this new aortic channel. But, currently there is no long-term follow-up of this approach.

15. Complications of surgery for ATAD

Based on the NORCAAD registry [50].

1. Bleeding
   i. Major bleeding –39 %
   ii. Reoperation for bleeding 22%.
   iii. Cardiac tamponade –15%
2. Neurological
   i. Stroke 20%.
   ii. Coma 11%.
   iii. Transient ischemic attack 5%.
3. Infections:
   i. Sepsis 10%.
   ii. Deep sternal wound infections 2%.
   iii. Pneumonia 19%
4. Renal
   i. Acute kidney injury 39%.
   ii. Renal replacement therapy 12%
5. Malperfusion
   i. Mesenteric ischemia 6%.
   ii. Myocardial infarction 6%.
   iii. Limb ischemia requiring surgery 4%

6. Reoperations of the aorta

    i. Proximal reoperation.

    ii. 1 year 0.8%.

    iii. 5 years 2.1%

7. Distal reoperations.

    i. year 0.8%

    ii. 5 years 4.3%

Bleeding is one of the most feared complication from a surgeon's point of view. When blood comes in contact with subendothelial tissue of false lumen, it leads to a coagulopathy. Consumption of coagulation factors and fibrinolysis leads to disseminated intravascular coagulation. Activation and consumption of platelets also contributes to mortality [51]. Patients with pre-operative cardiac mal-perfusion was found to be associated with 30-day mortality of 33% (47). Pre-operative cerebral malperfusion is associated with three-fold increase in risk of stroke. Post-operative stroke and coma occurred in 10–15% and 3–9% patients respectively in one series [46]. Acute kidney injury may occur in 40–55% [50].

16. Long-term follow-up

Long-term post-operative survival in recent years at 5, 10 and 30 years is 84–85, 64–68, and 38%, respectively [52]. Health-related quality of life is lower compared to the general population. There is 32% incidence of depression and post-traumatic stress disorder [53]. Over 50% patients have resistant hypertension on follow-up.

As per the EACTS/ESC 2014 guidelines, a follow-up CT-scan of the aorta is recommended at 1, 6 and 12 months and annually thereafter [54]. There are no recommendations specific to the aortic valve or aortic regurgitation for follow-up. To follow general guidelines, one can perform follow-up echocardiography every 1–2 years for mild regurgitation and annually for moderate and asymptomatic severe regurgitation [55].

17. Conclusion

Type A Aortic dissection is an emergency requiring timely surgical intervention. With improved imaging techniques, an accurate diagnosis can now be made. Open surgical repair techniques have given good long-term results. Endovascular intervention is an emerging less invasive option which can be combined with a surgical approach to give excellent long-term results.

Abbreviations

TAAD	type A aortic dissection
aSCP	antegrade selective cerebral perfusion
RCP	retrograde cerebral perfusion

Author details

Imran Khan[1*], Prashant Joshi[2], Adrian W. Pick[2] and Julian A. Smith[2]

1 Department of Cardiothoracic Surgery, Royal North Shore Hospital, Sydney, Australia

2 Department of Cardiothoracic Surgery, Monash Medical Centre, Melbourne, Australia

*Address all correspondence to: imran_khan261@yahoo.com

References

[1] Golledge J, Eagle KA. Acute aortic dissection. Lancet. 2008;**372**:55-66

[2] Olsson C, Thelin S, Stahle E, Ekbon A, Granath F. Thoracic aortic aneurysm and dissection: Increasing prevalence and improved outcomes reported in a nationwide population based study of more than 14000 cases from 1987 to 2002. Circulation. 2006;**114**:2611-2618

[3] Mehta RH, Manfredini R, Hassan F, et al. Chronological patterns of acute aortic dissection. Circulation. 2002;**106**:1110-1115

[4] DeBakey ME, McCollum CH, Crawford ES, et al. Dissection and dissecting aneurysms of the aorta: Twenty year follow up of five hundred twenty seven patients treated surgically. Surgery. 1982;**92**(6):1118-1134

[5] Nienaber CA, Clough RE. Management of acute aortic dissection. Lancet. 2015;**385**(9970):800-811

[6] Augoustides JG, Szeto WY, Desai ND, et al. Classification of acute type A dissection: Focus on clinical presentation and extent. European Journal of Cardiothoracic Surgery. 2011;**39**(4):519-522

[7] Geirsson A, Aklsson A, Franco-Cereceda A, et al. The Nordic consortium for acute type A aortic dissection (NORCAAD): Objectives and design. Scandinavian Cardiovascular Journal. 2016;**50**(5-6):334-340

[8] Landenhed M, Engstrom G, Gottsater A, et al. Risk profiles for aortic dissection and ruptured or surgically treated aneurysms: A prospective cohort study. Journal of the American Heart Association. 2015;**4**(1):e-1513

[9] Wojnarski CM, Svenson LG, Roselli EE, et al. Aortic dissection in patients with bicuspid aortic valve—Associated aneurysms. The Annals of Thoracic Surgery. 2015 Nov;**100**(5):1666-1674

[10] Geirsson A, Shioda K, Olsson C, et al. Differential outcomes of open and clamp-on distal anastomoses techniques in acute type A aortic dissection. The Journal of Thoracic and Cardiovascular Surgery. 2019;**157**:1750-1758

[11] Elsayed RS, Cohen RG, Fleischman F, et al. Acute type A aortic dissection. Cardiology Clinics. 2017;**35**(3):331-345

[12] Czerny H, Schoenhoff F, Etz C, et al. The impact of pre-operative malperfusion on outcome in acute type A aortic dissection: Results from the GERAADA registry. Journal of the American College of Cardiology. 2015;**65**(24):2628-2635

[13] Rogers AM, Hermann LK, Booher AM, Nienebar CA, Williams DM, Kazerooni EA, et al. Sensitivity of the aortic dissection risk score, a novel guideline based tool for identification of acute aortic dissection at initial presentation: Results from the international registry of acute aortic dissection. Circulation. 2011;**123**:2213-2218

[14] Hagan PG, Ninebar CA, Isselbacher EM, Bruckman D, Karavite DJ, Russman PL, et al. The international registry of acute aortic dissection (IRAD): New insights into an old disease. JAMA. 2000;**283**:897-903

[15] Rogers IS, Banerji D, Siegel EL, et al. Usefulness of comprehensive cardiothoracic computed tomography in the evaluation of acute undifferentiated chest discomfort in the emergency department (CAPTURE). The American Journal of Cardiology. 2011;**107**(5):643-650

[16] Meredith EL, Masani ND. Echocardiography in the emergency assessment of acute aortic syndromes. European Journal of Echocardiography. 2009;**10**(1):131-139

[17] Nienehar CA, Clough RE, Sakalikhson N, et al. Aortic dissection. Nature Reviews. Disease Primers. 2016;**2**:16071

[18] Rylski B. Endovascular repair of acute type A aortic dissection. We have the rechnology but where is the courage? Interactive Cardiovascular and Thoracic Surgery. 2017;**25**:501-502

[19] Creswell LL, Kouchoukos NT, Cox JL, Rosenbloom M. Coronary artery disease in patients with type A aortic dissection. The Annals of Thoracic Surgery. 1995;**59**:585-590

[20] Erbel R, Alfonso F, Boileau C, Dirsch O, Eber B, Haverick A, et al. Diagnosis and management of aortic dissection. European Heart Journal. 2001;**22**:1642-1681

[21] Carl M, Alms A, Braun J, Dougas A, Erl J, Goetz A, et al. S3 guidelines for intensive care in cardiac surgery patients: hemodynamic monitoring and cardiocirculatory system. German Medical Science. 2010;**8**:Doc 12

[22] Tsiouris A, Elkinavy S, Ziganshin BA, Elefteriades JA. Open Seldinger guided femoral artery cannulation technique for thoracic aortic surgery. The Annals of Thoracic Surgery. 2016;**101**:2231-2235

[23] Valentine RJ, Wind G. Anatomic Exposures in Vascular Surgery. Philadelphia: Lippincott Wlliams and Williams; 2003

[24] Ogino H, Sasaki H, Minatoya K, Matsuda H, Tauaka H, Watannki H, et al. Evolving arch surgery using integrated antegrade selective cerebral perfusion: Impact of axillary artery perfusion. Journal of Thoracic and Cadiovascualr Surgery. 2008;**136**: 641-648

[25] Sabik JF, Lytle BW, McCartht PM, Cosgrove DM. Axillary artery: An alternative site of arterial cannulation for patients with extensive aortic and peripheral vascular disease. The Journal of Thoracic and Cardiovascular Surgery. 1995;**109**:885-890

[26] Pasic M, Schubel J, Buer M, Yankah C, Kuppe M, et al. Cannulation of right axillary artery for surgery of acute type A aortic dissection. European Journal of Cardio-Thoracic Surgery. 2003;**24**:231-235

[27] Sabashnikov A, Heinen S, Deppe AC, Zeriouh M, Weymann A, et al. Axillary or aortic cannulation for aortic repair in patients with stanford a dissection? The Annals of Thoracic Surgery. 2016;**102**(3):787-794

[28] McCullough JN, Zhang N, Reich DL, et al. Cerebral metabolic suppression during hypothermic circulatory arrest in humans. The Annals of Thoracic Surgery. 1999;**67**:1895-1899

[29] Ueda Y. A reappraisal of retrograde cerebral perfusion. Annals of Cardiothoracic Surgery. 2013;**2**(3):316-325. DOI: 10.3978/j.issn.2225-319X.2013.01.02

[30] Reich DL, Uysal S, Ergin MA, et al. Retrograde cerebral perfusion during thoracic aortic surgery and late neuropsychological dysfunction. European Journal of Cardio-Thoracic Surgery. 2001;**19**:594-600

[31] Liebeskind DS. Collateral circulation. Stroke. 2003;**34**:2279-2284

[32] Bachet J, Guilnet D, Goudot B, Delentdecker P, Brodaty D, et al. Antegrade cerebral perfusion with cold blood: A 13 year experience. The Annals of Thoracic Surgery. 1999;**67**(6):1874-1878

[33] Kazui T. Total arch replacement with separated graft technique and selective antegrade cerebral perfusion. Annals of Cardiothoracic Surgery. 2013;**2**(3):353-357

[34] Griepp RB. Cerebral protection during aortic arch surgery. The Journal of Thoracic and Cardiovascular Surgery. 2001;**121**:425-427

[35] Malvindi PG, Scrascia G, Vitale N. Is unilateral antegrade cerebral perfusion equivalent to bilateral cerebral perfusion for patients undergoing arch surgery? Interactive Cradiovascualr and Thoracic Surgery. 2008;**7**:891-897

[36] Kruger T, Weigang E, Hoffmann I, Blettner M, Aebert H, GERAADA INVESTIGATORS. Cerebral protection during surgery for acute aortic dissection type A: Results of the German registry for acute aortic dissection type A (GERAADA). European Journal of Cardio-Thoracic Surgery. 2011;**40**:435-440

[37] Di Eusanio M, Trimarchi S, Peterson MD, et al. Root replacement surgery versus more conservative management during type A acute aortic dissection repair. The Annals of Thoracic Surgery. 2014;**98**:2078-2084

[38] Varrica A, Satriano A, de Vincentiis C, Biondi A, Trimarchi S, et al. Bentall operation in 375 patients: Long-term results and predictors of death. The Journal of Heart Valve Disease. 2014 Jan;**23**(1):127-134

[39] Leshnower BG, Myung RJ, McPherson L, et al. Midterm results of David V valve sparing aortic root replacement in acute type A aortic dissection. Annals of Thoarcic Surgery. 2015;**99**:795-800

[40] Park KH, Lim C, Choi JH, et al. Midterm change of descending aortic false lumen after repair of acute type A dissection. The Annals of Thoracic Surgery. 2009;**87**:103-108

[41] Rylski B, Bavaria JE, Milewski RK, et al. Long term results of neomedia sinus valsalva repair in 489 patients with type A aortic dissection. Annals of Thoarcic Surgery. 2014;**98**:582-588

[42] Kruger T, Weigang E, Hoffman I, Blettner M, Aebert H, GERAADA INVESTIGATORS. Cerebral protection during surgery for acute aortic dissection type A: Results of the German registry for acute aortic dissection type A (GERAADA). Circulation. 2011;**124**:434-443

[43] Halstead JC, Meier M, Etz C, Spielvogel D, Bodian C, Wurm M, et al. The fate of the distal aorta after repair of acute type A aortic dissection. The Journal of Thoracic and Cardiovascular Surgery. 2007;**133**:127-135

[44] Kim JB, Chung CH, Moon DH, et al. Total arch repair versus hemiarch repair in the management of acute DeBakey type I aortic dissection. European Journal of Cardio-Thoracic Surgery. 2011;**40**:881-887

[45] Weigang E, Conzelmann L, Kallenbach K, et al. German registry for acute aortic dissection type a (GERAADA)-lessons learned from the registry. The Thoracic and Cardiovascular Surgeon. 2010;**58**:154-158

[46] Kazui T, Yamashita K, Washiyama N, et al. Impact of an aggressive surgical approach on surgical outcome in type A aortic dissection. The Annals of Thoracic Surgery. 2002;**74**:S1844-S1847

[47] Uchida N, Shibamura H, Katyama A, et al. Operative strategy for acute type a aortic dissection: Ascending aortic or Hemiarch versus Total arch replacement with frozen elephant trunk. The Annals of Thoracic Surgery. 2009;**87**:773-777

[48] Cifani N, Proietta M, Tritapepe L, Die Gioia C, Ferri L, Taurino M, et al. Stanford—A acute aortic dissection,

inflammation and metalloproteinases: A review. Annals of Medicine. 2015;**45**:441-446

[49] Matalanis G, Ips S. A new paradigm in the management of acute type A aortic dissection: Total aortic repair. The Journal of Thoracic and Cardiovascular Surgery. 2019;**157**(1):3-11

[50] Zindovic I, Gudbjartsson T, Ahlsson A, et al. Malperfusion in acute type A aortic dissection: An update from the Nordic Consortium for acute type A aortic dissection. The Journal of Thoracic and Cardiovascular Surgery. 2019;**157**:1324.e6-1336.e6

[51] Cate JW, Timers H, Becker AE. Coagulopathy in ruptured or dissecting aortic aneurysms. The American Journal of Medicine. 1975;**59**(2):171-176

[52] Pan E, Kyoto V, Savunen T, et al. Earrly and late outcomes after open ascending aortic surgery: 47 year experience in a single centre. Heart and Vessels. 2018;**33**(4):427-433

[53] Endlich M, Hamiko M, Gestrich C, et al. Long term outcome and quality of life in aortic type A dissection survivors. The Journal of Thoracic and Cardiovascular Surgery. 2016;**64**:91-99

[54] Hiratzka LF, Bakris GL, Beckman JA, et al. ACCF/AHA/AATS/ACR/ASA/SCA/SCAI/SIR/STS/SVM Guidelines for the diagnosis and management of patients with thoracic aortic disease. A Report of the American College of Cardiology Foundation/American Heart Association Task Force on Practice Guidelines, American Association for Thoracic Surgery, American College of Radiology, American Stroke Association, Society of Cardiovascular Anesthesiologists, Society for Cardiovascular Angiography and Interventions, Society of Interventional Radiology, Society of Thoracic Surgeons, and Society for Vascular Medicine. Journal of the American College of Cardiology. 2010, 2010;**55**(14):e27-e129

[55] Baumgartner H, Falk V, Bax JJ, et al. 2017 ESC/EACTS guidelines for the management of valvular heart disease. European Heart Journal. 2017;**38**(36):2739-2791

Chapter 5

Transcatheter Treatment of Aortic Stenosis and Regurgitation

Zhang Haibo and Meng Xu

Abstract

Since the successful application of transcatheter aortic valve implantation (TAVI) in 2002, the interventional treatment of valvular heart disease has developed rapidly. The interventional treatment of aortic valve stenosis or insufficiency has been more mature, and many new-generation TAVI valves have been developed. The recommended level of TAVI technology in the European and American heart valve disease guidelines has increased year by year. In 2019, the multi-center randomized controlled study on patients with low-risk aortic stenosis and conventional aortic valve replacement also showed the advantages of interventional treatment technology, such as small trauma, fast recovery and less complications, and better hemodynamics, which greatly promoted the development of TAVI technology.

Keywords: transcatheter aortic valve implantation, aortic valve stenosis, aortic valve regurgitation, heart team, heart valve disease

1. Introduction

Aortic valve disease is common in the elderly people. In clinical practice, many elderly patients, as well as patients with other organ dysfunctions, cannot tolerate the valve replacement surgery of open chest with cardiopulmonary bypass. Transcatheter aortic valve implantation (TAVI) technology can complete valve replacement without thoracotomy, cardiac arrest, and cardiopulmonary bypass. Its advantages are obvious. This chapter will review the research and development history of TAVIi technology and different design features of TAVI valve, especially the application effect of China-designed TAVI valves in China. What's more, TAVI technology brings not only technological innovation, but also a new team cooperation mode for disease treatment, which can better provide heart valve disease patients with higher quality and safer tsreatment. Finally, in addition to the aortic stenosis, earliest indications of TAVI, it can also be used for the treatment of aortic valve regurgitation. The new generation of TAVI valve has a unique design helpful in leaflets fixation and clamping, which can complete the interventional treatment easily.

2. The development history of TAVI techniques

Aortic valve stenosis is a common cardiovascular disease. In western countries, the incidence is about 2.0% in people aged ≥65 and 4.0% in people aged ≥85, which is second only to hypertension and coronary heart disease [1–3]. As early as the 1960s, researchers imitated vascular stents to treat aortic insufficiency by placing metal stents, but these designs stopped after animal trials because of many problems in hemodynamics, postoperative anticoagulation, and so on. Among the non-operative interventional techniques for early aortic stenosis, only balloon dilatation (balloon aortic valvuloplasty, BAV) can be approved for clinical use. The technique, pioneered by Alain Cribier in 1985, is mainly used in patients with severe aortic stenosis who cannot be operated by routine open heart surgery. Many patients can improve short- and medium-term results, but the 1-year recurrence rate can be as high as 80% [4, 5]. However, due to the urgent need for high-risk patients undergoing thoracotomy, more than 1500 patients with severe aortic stenosis have received this treatment.

In the course of development since then, the stent interventional therapy of coronary artery disease has given a lot of revelation to the interventional therapy of valvular disease. In February 1989, at a medical conference in Phoenix City, USA, after listening to an academic report on coronary intervention stents, Sweden doctor Henning R. Andersen had a whim: if calcified coronary artery stenosis can be solved with metal stents, can aortic valve stenosis be done in a similar way? The first metal stent material that Andersen tried was the most commonly used sternal fixation wire in cardiac surgery, which was molded into a U-shaped structure in order to achieve a telescopic purpose. In May 1989, the prototype conceptual system of TAVI surgery emerged. From idea to feasibility verification, it took Andersen only two and a half months to revolutionize the diagnosis and treatment of aortic valve disease in the twenty-first century. The technology of transcatheter aortic valve implantation was born. Finally, in 1995, the famous patent for Andersen interventional valve was approved in the United States [6].

In the early stage after the feasibility verification of TAVI technology, it went through a long and difficult road of not being recognized. Andersen submitted the completed paper to the *Journal of the American College of Cardiology* (in 1990, when the influence factor of JACC was 5.9), but the reply was that "there is no advantage of this study to be published in JACC magazine." (It has too low priority for publication in JACC). Subsequently, the improved article in 1991 was submitted to Circulation (then impact factor 9.0), and the reply was still rejected. In 1992, at the European Heart annual meeting and the American Heart Association (AHA) annual meeting, the TAVI technology research report submitted by Andersen was arranged to be presented in a poster, and no one paid attention to it.

After that, the first TAVI animal experimental operation was successful, which confirmed the feasibility of the design concept. The article on animal experiments was published in European Heart Journal in 1992 [6]. TAVI technology has finally begun to attract attention, and other similar stent valve designs with animal studies have also begun to emerge. Alain Cribier's team also conducted in-depth research on this technology in 1993 and 1994, including the research and development of balloon-dilated valve stents, selection of stent materials, length and shape design considerations, and so on. However, throughout the 1990s, there was still no breakthrough in TAVI technology due to the high failure rate in animal experiments and the engineering and technical bottleneck in the manufacture of stent valves.

In 2000, Philipp Bonhoeffer and others first tried to use bovine jugular vein to make valve into platinum metal stent and then loaded it on the balloon delivery system to carry out sheep pulmonary valve replacement. The valve also successfully completed the first human pulmonary valve implantation in the same year [7]. However, there are great defects in the follow-up funding and design, which leads to the gradual cessation of the technology research.

Alain Cribier's team continued the study of balloon dilatation of the stent valve, testing the stainless steel stent in 12 aortic valve stenosis specimens obtained from human surgery, confirming that the stent could open the natural valve repeatedly, regardless of the valve's calcification. And they concluded the ideal height of the stent may be 14–16 mm, which can avoid blocking the coronary opening and interventricular septum or affecting the anterior leaflet of the mitral valve. Then Percutaneous Valve Technologies, a PVT company led by Alain Cribier, was founded in 1999 with the help of investors and medical valve companies. The engineer R&D team of the Israeli subsidiary officially began the design and development of the interventional valve. After a great deal of laboratory work, the first TAVI valve model (balloon dilatation) was born soon [8]. On April 16, 2002, Alain Cribier successfully completed the world's first TAVI operation with Cribier-Edwards interventional valve in Lyon, France, which opened the prelude to the development of TAVI technology. Since then, 40 operations have been completed [9]. Edwards acquired PVT for $150 million after an initial investment in 2003.

Alain Cribier used the transfemoral vein method to enter the aortic valve for TAVI. John Webb of Canada collaborated with Edwards to develop retrograde arterial implantation. The technique has a deflectable sheath that can easily pass through the aortic arch and the narrowed valve orifice [10]. John Webb and his colleagues also performed the first transapical valve implantation [11]. Walther et al. promoted the number of cases of TAVI via Edwards' apical approach as an easier way to implant the valve [12].

After Jacques Seguin founded CoreValve in the United States in 2001, Eberhard Grube carried out the first clinical implantation of CoreValve valve in 2005 after previous animal experiments [13]. The results proved the feasibility of using self-expanding valve for TAVI. At the ACC meeting in 2006, Grube reported the first group of 14 patients who underwent TAVI with self-expanding CoreValve valves. At that time, only nine of these patients had no adverse cardiac events in the first 2 weeks. The device can be implanted via femoral artery approach. The CoreValve valve has been continuously improved since then, and the company was acquired by Medtronic in February 2009. Since then, the CoreValve valve has been replaced by a series of Evolut valves. In 2007, the Edwards SAPIEN valve and CoreValve valve first entered the European market and obtained CE approval. Since 2012, they have been approved by the FDA in the United States for surgical high-risk patients with aortic valve stenosis. Since then, the technology has developed by leaps and bounds, and research centers in Europe and the United States have successfully carried out more than 20 clinical multicenter randomized controlled trials, proving the safety and effectiveness of TAVI technology.

This is an epoch-making minimally invasive surgical technique that does not require thoracotomy and extracorporeal circulation or cardiac arrest. A large number of expert consensus and guidelines have been issued, and the recommendation level of TAVI has been gradually improved. Andersen successfully performed TAVI surgery on his father in 2011, and he defined this time as the end of a perfect cycle of his research.

In the European 2012 guidelines, TAVI candidates are limited to surgical high-risk patients and require the presence of surgeons and the heart team (heart team) to make decisions [14]. Through the safety and effectiveness of TAVI technology with the rapid development of the new generation of valve and technical experience, many clinical research results continue to get good results, and the recommendation level of TAVI in European and American valvular disease guidelines is getting higher and higher. In 2010, the PARTNER 1B study pointed out that although TAVI has incidence of massive hemorrhage and vascular complications in patients with inoperable aortic valve stenosis, the incidence of all-cause mortality, readmission and cardiac symptoms is significantly lower than that of standard treatment [15]. The results of 5-year follow-up of PARTNER IB (inoperable) were released at the 2014 Annual Meeting of Transcatheter Cardiovascular Therapeautics (TCT), suggesting that compared with standard treatment, TAVI had significant benefits in terms of all-cause death rate (71.8%: 93.6%), cardiovascular death (57.3%: 85.9%), readmission rate (47.6%: 87.3%), and improvement of cardiac function (III: IV = 14.3%: 40%). In 2016, the PARTNER 2 study turned to the medium-risk population, confirming that the mortality, disability, and stroke incidence of TAVI and surgical surgery was similar [16]. The PARTNER III study and the EVOLUTE study published similar results in 2019. In these randomized controlled study of patients with low-risk aortic valve stenosis, whether it is balloon-expandable valve or self-expanding valve, the mortality and complication rate of TAVI group is better than that of conventional thoracotomy group. As a result, the United States and European Drug Regulatory agencies have extended the use of TAVI to patients with low-risk aortic stenosis since 2019 [17, 18].

In 2015, about 40,000 patients in Europe received TAVI treatment, and that number will rise to 60,000 in 2020. The number of patients with TAVI indications in Europe is expected to exceed 114,000/year, and if extended to low-risk patients, it can increase to 177,000/year. In France, 1600 and 8000 patients were treated with TAVI in 2010 and 2015, respectively, and the figure is expected to reach 10,000 in 2016. Germany receives TAVI treatment for every 1 million residents, which has the highest TAVI implementation rate in Europe. There were more than 15,000 cases in Germany in 2016, three times as many as in 2011. The number of valve replacement cases in routine surgery remained relatively stable, with no less than 10,000 cases per year. In developed countries such as Germany (2013) and the United States (2019), the number of TAVI surgeries has exceeded that of conventional thoracotomy aortic valve replacement, and the gap is still widening. A total of more than 400,000 TAVI operations have been completed worldwide.

In 2018, Durko et al. used Monte Carlo mathematical model combined with 37 clinical studies of 26,402 cases of severe aortic valve stenosis to predict the number of patients with TAVI indications each year in Europe and the United States. In patients over 65 years old, the incidence of severe aortic stenosis was 4.4‰ per year. 68.3% patients with severe aortic stenosis had related symptoms. Despite severe symptoms of aortic stenosis, 41.6% did not undergo surgical aortic valve replacement. Of the nonsurgical patients, 61.7% received TAVI treatment. This model predicts 114,757 European and 58,556 North American TAVI candidates each year. The conclusion is that there are currently about 180,000 patients a year in the European Union and North America who can be considered potential candidates for TAVI. If the indications for TAVI are extended to low-risk patients, this number may increase to 270,000. These findings have a significant impact on healthcare resource planning in 29 countries [19].

The European Valve observation registration study (EURObservational Research Programme VHD II) conducted a survey at 22 centers in 28 countries to show changes in the structure of heart valve patients and their impact on clinical treatment. 7247 patients with VHD (including 4483 inpatients and 2764 outpatients) were enrolled in the study. Compared with a similar survey conducted in 2005, the latest survey in 2019 showed that the actual treatment strategies of patients with aortic valve disease were more in-line with the guidelines and the proportion of transcatheter therapy was gradually increasing (39% of aortic stenosis and 17% of mitral regurgitation) [20].

The SAPIEN 3 valve is the third generation in the SAPIEN series of valves developed by Edwards. The valve stent contains an outward reflexed skirt, which can prevent perivalvular leakage. The delivery system as a whole becomes smaller, shrinking to 14F (16F for 29 mm valves). At the same time, the conveying system has good controllability, so that the near-center section of the conveying system can be bent and maintain better coaxiality. The SAPIEN 3 Ultra is an improved and upgraded version of the SAPIEN 3 valve system, and a 14F sheath can be used for all sizes of valves [21]. Centera is a self-expanding valve developed by Edwards Corporation. This valve is quite different from Medtronic's self-expanding valve. Its nickel-titanium stent is short, similar to a balloon-expandable valve, using a bovine pericardial valve. There is a metal wire at the waist of the stent, which can be tightened to retract the valve so that it can be retrieved. The conveying system is 14F, which can be bent to ensure the release with good coaxiality. The electric release handle makes the release easier, and the valve can be released by a single operator. Centera valve design combines the characteristics of self-expandable stents (recyclable stents with good deformability) and ball-expanded stents (short stents and low incidence of pacemakers) [22].

The Evolut R valve is an upgraded version of the Medtronic CoreValve valve. The valve enhances the radial force at the annulus level, and the lower end of the skirt extends downward to prevent perivalvular leakage. The valve stent is shorter, so that the coaxial line of the stent is better after release. The shape of the stent is more straight and cylindrical. More importantly, a nickel-titanium casing is arranged at the near end of the delivery system, and before the valve stent is completely released, the valve can be pulled back to the nickel-titanium casing to achieve retrieved; thus the position of the valve can be readjusted. On the basis of Evolut R, Evolut pro wrapped a pericardial patch around the lower segment of the stent to reduce the incidence of perivalvular leakage and pacemaker implantation [23–25].

The Lotus Edge valve is a product developed by Boston Science Co., Ltd., which is an upgraded version of the Lotus valve. The Lotus valve stent is made of Ni-Ti alloy. The diameter of the short axis of the stent can be shortened after lengthening longitudinally, so as to achieve the purpose of recycling. The lower part of the device has an adaptive sealing ring, which can reduce the incidence of perivalvular regurgitation. Lotus Edge retains the advantages of full retrieved valve of Lotus, prevention of perivalvular leakage, early valvular work, and so on. At the same time, the delivery system is improved to make it softer and more curved. More important is the implantation depth protection technology to prevent the valve from entering the outflow tract too deep, thus reducing the incidence of conduction block. In previous clinical trials, the implantation rate of Lotus pacemakers was as high as 35.5% and was later withdrawn from the market. Lotus Edge is expected to reduce the pacemaker implantation rate compared with Lotus. In April 2019, the Lotus Edge valve was approved for sale by the FDA in the United States [26].

ACCURATE neo is a self-expanding valve implanted via artery, and it is also a design of Ni-Ti alloy stent and supra-annular valve. Its unique design lies in that it contains an anchoring device and can be positioned automatically. The release of the valve is different from that of other self-expanding valves. Generally, the self-expanding valve first releases the proximal end and then releases the distal end. During the ACCURATE neo release procedure, the distal end is first released, the anchoring device exposed, and the valve stent is leaded down to the autologous aortic annulus level and then the proximal part is released. It also contains the outer edge of the skirt to prevent the valve from leaking. The distal stent grid has a large aperture and does not interfere with percutaneous coronary intervention after valve implantation. The lower part of the stent is covered by the inner layer and the outer layer of the pericardium to prevent perivalvular leakage. Its delivery system is equivalent to 15F. In the latest large randomized controlled study, 739 patients (mean age 82.8 years, STS score 3.5%) were randomly divided into two groups: ACCURATE neo valve 367 cases and SAPIEN 3 valve 364 cases. The main end point of ACCURATE neo 30 days and SAPIEN 3 did not achieve non-inferiority (24% vs. 16% personality 0.42). Although there was no difference in 30-day mortality (2 vs. 1%) and stroke (2 vs. 3%) between the two groups, the incidence of acute renal injury (3% vs. 1%) and moderate perivalvular leakage (9 vs. 3%) was higher in the ACCURATE neo group [27].

The JenaValve valve is specially designed [28, 29]. The stent valve with three fixed keys is implanted through the apical approach. TF-JenaValve is the new version of JenaValve via the femoral artery. The JenaValve is a short stent with a large mesh hole at the upper end, which is beneficial to the introduction of the coronary artery. The outer edge of the stent contains three anchoring parts, which can prevent the stent from being fixed to the bottom of the three aortic sinuses. The artificial valve is designed for supra-annular valve. The JenaValve deployment first releases the proximal anchoring device, then pushes it to the autologous aortic valve annulus, automatically locates and gets stuck, then releases the proximal stent, and finally releases the distal connecting device. The delivery system of TF-JenaValve is 18F, which has a bending function to ensure the coaxiality of the release valve and the aortic valve annulus. The design of the JenaValve with a fixed key makes it possible to treat aortic regurgitation and patients with low coronary artery openings. This is similar to the Chinese domestic J-Valve.

The design of the Engager valve produced by Medtronic is similar to that of the JenaValve valve. It is also a valve implanted through the apical approach. By placing the control arm with anatomical positioning function at the root of the aortic sinus, the valve stent can be positioned accurately, and the complications can be reduced [30, 31].

3. The development of TAVI technology in China

According to incomplete statistics, China has a total population of 1.4 billion, including 44.8 million elderly people over the age of 75 (3.4%), and about 1.5 million patients (3.4%) with severe aortic valve stenosis, including about 0.2 million high-risk patients and 0.3 million moderate-risk patients. A single-center survey led by Gao Runlin showed that among the 139,496 patients examined by echocardiography from January 2010 to December 2015, the detection rate of severe mitral regurgitation was the highest (0.68%). This was followed by mitral stenosis (0.38%), aortic stenosis (0.28%), and aortic regurgitation (0.27%) [32]. From January 2009 to December 2013, Liu et al. investigated 19,428 patients with abnormal valvular structure or function in Guangdong People's Hospital, of which 13,549 (69.7%) were relatively certain to be valvular heart disease through clinical data, patient characteristics, and echocardiography. Among these patients, rheumatic heart disease accounted for 37.0%, and congenital valvular disease accounted for 13.9%. Degenerative valvular disease accounted for 11.5%, ischemic valvular disease accounted for 12.7%, infectious valvular disease accounted for 3.1%, and autoimmune-mediated valvular disease accounted for 0.7%. In 5 years, rheumatic heart disease decreased from 42.8% in 2009 to 32.8% in 2013 ($P < 0.001$), while degenerative valvular heart disease increased from 8.8% to 14.5% ($P < 0.001$), ischemic valvular disease increased from 9.2% to 11.3% ($P = 0.003$), and congenital valvular disease increased from 9.0% to 12.3% ($P < 0.001$). The prevalence of degenerative valvular disease is dominant in patients over 65 years old much more than rheumatic valvular disease [33]. The level of medical treatment level in different regions of China is uneven, and the evaluation of surgical risks and taboos is different from that of foreign countries. A 20-year review of data from Changhai Hospital affiliated to the Second Military Medical University in Shanghai showed that among the 6300 patients who underwent valve replacement of the left heart system, only 2.0% were over 70 years old, and the maximum age was 79 years old [34]. Another study included 521 consecutive valve surgery patients, of whom 53 (10%) were assessed to be at the highest risk before operation, with an average STS score of only 3.25 [35].

In 2002, the world's first TAVI operation was completed; in 2010, the first China TAVI operation was completed (GE Junbo, Zhongshan Hospital) [36].

In 2012, China's first independent intellectual property valve product Venus A began clinical trials; 7 cases were completed nationwide.

In 2015, GE Junbo, Wang Jianan, and other organizations have reached the consensus of Chinese experts on transcatheter aortic valve replacement [37].

In 2017, the Venus A valve via the femoral artery and the J-Valve valve via the apical approach were officially approved and put on the market, marking a new era of interventional therapy for valvular heart disease in China. In 2017, the United States issued the consensus of experts on the clinical decision-making path of transcatheter aortic valve replacement for adult aortic valve stenosis [38].

In 2018, more than 1000 TAVI operations were completed nationwide in China. GE Junbo and Wang Jianan [39] published the Chinese expert consensus on transcatheter aortic valve replacement team construction and operation standard. Wu Yongjian and others issued the clinical pathway of transcatheter aortic valve implantation in China [40]. Zhang Yun and others organized the China expert consensus on perioperative echocardiographic examination of transcatheter aortic valve implantation [41]. Cheng Weiping and Li Lihuan organized the Chinese anesthesia expert consensus on TAVR surgery clinical Ppathway Mmanagement [42]. Wang Chunsheng and others published the Chinese transcatheter aortic valve implantation (TAVI) multidisciplinary expert consensus [43]. Xu Zhiyun and Lu Fanglin started the interventional tricuspid valve clinical trials with LUX valve. Hu Shengshou and Meng Xu led the mitral stitch technique of trans-apical artificial chordae tendineae implantation to begin clinical trials. GE Junbo and Zhou Daxin led the trans-apical mitral valve double-hole valve clamp technique to begin clinical trials.

In 2019, the VitaFlow valve (via the femoral artery) was approved to be put on the Chinese market. 2000 TAVI operations were performed by cardiologists and surgeons all over the country. Xu et al. led the establishment of the Academic Committee on Interventional Therapy of Cardiac Valvular Disease and published the expert consensus on the responsibilities and requirements of cardiac surgeons in cardiac team Building [44]. Haibo and others developed innovation with J-Valve valve in valve techniques for mitral and tricuspid tissue valve deterioration [45]. Both Edwards SAPIEN valve and domestic Taurus valve have completed clinical trials and are expected to be on the market within 2 years. Runlin et al. released good 5-year follow-up results of Venus A valve and J-Valve valve, which showed that their safety and effectiveness had been verified in the medium and long term.

At present, a total of 150 centers in China have the ability to carry out TAVI surgery, of which there are about 10 units; the cumulative number of TAVI cases is more than 100 cases. Different from Europe and the United States, Chinese patients with bicuspid aortic valve are in the majority, with more severe calcification, more weakness in elderly patients, and more complications when they see a doctor later. And at present, there are obvious differences in TAVI experience and team construction among different centers in China, most of which are in the initial stage of the learning curve, with both opportunities and challenges. With the introduction of a new generation of valves into clinical practice, the success rate of TAVI in various centers in China will continue to improve, and more clinical experience needs to be accumulated. In the aspect of image evaluation, combined with the individual characteristics of the Chinese population, the multiplane valvular three dimentional measurement technique proposed by Wu Yongjian of Fuwai Hospital, the small balloon measurement method put forward by the Zhongshan Hospital affiliated to Fudan University, and the sequential balloon measurement strategy put forward by Wang Jianan of the Second Affiliated Hospital of Zhejiang University Medical College. The optimized measurement technology of optimal reshaping put forward by Chen Mao of West China Hospital of Sichuan University and the concept of effective annular diameter and effective valve area of TAVI surgery put forward by Meng Xu and Zhang Haibo of Beijing Anzhen Hospital have made substantial contributions to the development of TAVI technology in China. The new generation of interventional valve represented by SAPIEN 3, Evolut R, and Centera has mainly improved the defects of early interventional valve, which is characterized by lower incidence of perivalvular leakage, retrievable, small delivery system, and automatic localization. At present, it is considered that the new interventional valve with the above two characteristics can be classified as the second-generation valve. In the research and development of the second-generation valve, China has gradually caught up with the pace of the world, and new-generation valves such as J-Valve developed by Suzhou Jiecheng Company, VitaFlow II valve developed by Shanghai Minimally Invasive Medical Devices Co., Ltd., and Venus A plus valve developed by Hangzhou Qiming Company have been implanted in the first patient one after another.

Venus A valve is the first TAVI valve on the market in China, which was implanted through the femoral artery. Up to October 2019, a total of more than 2000 Venus A TAVI operations have been performed in 142 centers in China. Among them, there were 19 centers with more than 20 TAVI cases, 16 centers with 10 cases, and 16 centers with less than 10 cases. The prospective multicenter observational study, which began in 2012 to evaluate the safety and efficacy of Venus A valve in the treatment of severe aortic valve stenosis, followed up patients with TAVI for 5 years. The results showed that the 5-year all-cause mortality rate was 20.8% and the cardiovascular mortality rate was 15.8%. The risk ratio of age > 85 years old was 1.47 [95%CI (1.12 ~ 2.00), P = 0.007], and the risk ratio of STS > 8 was 1.56 [95%CI (1.21–2.01), 0.033]. On March 29, 2019, at the China Interventional Cardiology Conference (CIT2019) in Beijing, Gao Runlin reported the results of a 5-year follow-up study with severe Venus A valve stenosis or severe regurgitation of 0 and moderate velocity increase or moderate regurgitation of less than 10%. The second generation interventional aortic valve system developed by Venus A plus has a retrievable function. Structurally, the valve release recyclable function is realized through innovative sheath design. The conveying system uses a 19F guide sheath. On the basis of the retrievable function, the Venus A pilot adds an adjustable bending function to ensure the coaxiality of the valve release. Qiming Venibri Valve is the world's first preinstalled TAVI valve, so that the valve can be used in the catheterization room, saving valuable time for critically ill patients to save lives [46].

VitaFlow II is a second-generation interventional aortic valve system developed by Shanghai Minimally Invasive Medical Devices Co., Ltd., which has the function of retrievable and anti-perivalvular leakage and belongs to the second-generation interventional aortic valve. VitaFlow II valve stent is the same generation of VitaFlow. Structurally, the valve release retrievable function is realized through innovative sheath design, that is, repositioning and rerelease. The design of the inner and outer tubes of the transportation system has an enhanced structure, which not only ensures the stability and accuracy of the release but also realizes the multidirectional bending function, so as to reduce the damage to blood vessels and reduce the probability of vascular complications. According to the characteristics of thinner femoral artery in Chinese elderly patients, the internal catheter sheath was set up to realize the integrated puncture function and reduce the vascular damage caused by the transportation system (equivalent to 16–18F sheath).

J-Valve is a self-expanding Ni-Ti stent, and there are three flexible fixed bond steel rings around the stent. Different from JenaValve in which fixed bond and Ni-Ti stent are welded, the J-Valve fixed bond and Ni-Ti stent are connected by string, which is beneficial for the movement of the fixed bond at the bottom of the sinus during release and better fit to the aortic sinus bottom. The conveying system is 18–22Fr with adjustable bending function. The valve release procedure is similar to that of JenaValve [47]. TF-J-Valve is the femoral artery version of J-Valve, and the valve design is basically the same as J-Valve. TF-J-Valve exploratory clinical trials are mainly conducted in Canada and have confirmed the technical feasibility [48].

4. Indications of TAVI in low-risk patients

Multiple death reasons analysis maintained by the National Center for Statistics from 2008 to 2017 [49] showed that the mortality rate due to aortic stenosis in the elderly in the United States has declined since 2013, while the number of TAVI hands has increased from 4627 in 2012 to nearly 35,000 in 2016. It is speculated that the observed death rate trend may be related to TAVI.

On March 17, 2019, in the American College of Cardiology (ACC) annual meeting, the low-risk patients TAVI studies PARTNER III and EVOLUT results were released, marking the comprehensive arrival of the TAVI era of severe aortic valve stenosis. Martin Leon of Columbia University Medical Center in New York officially released the results of PARTNER III study at the conference [17]. For low-risk patients with severe aortic stenosis, the incidence of 1-year death, infarction, and rehospitalization in patients with Edwards balloon-expandable TAVI valve implantation was significantly lower than that in patients undergoing open heart surgery. The study included 1000 patients from 71 centers, with an average age of 73 years and an average STS score of 1.9%. The main end point of the study was the compound end points, including 1-year death, infarction, and rehospitalization event rate. The results showed that the event rate of the main end point in the TAVI group was significantly lower than that in the surgical operation group (8.5% vs. 15.1%). The 30-day infarction rate (0.6 vs. 2.4%), infarction or death event rate (1.0% vs. 3.3%), and new atrial fibrillation rate (5.0% vs. 39.5%) in the TAVI group were significantly lower than those in the operation group. In addition, patients in the TAVI group had a shorter average hospital stay (3 days vs. 7 days) and a lower risk of a 30-day poor prognosis (death or low KCCQ score) (3.9% vs. 30.6%). There was no difference in the incidence of major vascular complications, permanent pacemaker implantation, and moderate or severe perivalvular leakage between the two groups.

The Evolut study included 1468 patients who underwent Medtronic self-expanding TAVI valves, of which 1403 underwent TAVI or surgery [18]. The average age of these patients was 74 years, and the main end point of the study was a 24-month complex event of death or crippling infarction. The incidence of major end point events at 24 months in the TAVI group was 5.3%, while that in the surgical group was 6.7%. The incidences of 30-day disabled infarction (0.5 vs. 1.7%), bleeding complications (2.4% vs. 7.5%), acute renal injury (0.9% vs. 2.8%), and atrial fibrillation (7.7% vs. 35.4%) in the TAVI group were significantly lower than those in the surgical group. However, moderate or severe perivalvular leakage (3.5 vs. 0.5%) and permanent pacemaker implantation rate (17.4% vs. 6.1%) were higher than those in the surgical group. At 1 year, the mortality rate in the TAVI group was 0.4%, while that in the surgical group was 1.2% (no significant).

The TAVI group had lower all-cause mortality and incidence of disabled infarction (but not statistically significant) (2.9% vs. 4.6%), significantly reduced crippling infarction (0.8% vs. 2.4%), and significantly reduced hospitalization for heart failure (3.2%vs. 6.5%). In addition, in the TAVI group, the transvalvular pressure difference was lower (8.6 mmHg vs. 11.2 mmHg), and the effective valve orifice area was larger (2.3 cm^2 vs. 2.0 cm^2) at 12 months. Despite the high proportion of perivalvular regurgitation after TAVI, only 22% of the patients received the third-generation valve. The new valve increases the edge of the skirt to reduce perivalvular leakage, so it is expected that the regurgitation rate will decrease as the new device utilization rate increases.

At present, there are about 60,000 TAVI operations in the United States every year. This may increase to 75,000 if patients at moderate risk received TAVI and to 100,000 or more if extended to low risk. The ultimate goal of TAVI surgery is that TAVI can be performed in all comers. It means no matter what the risk, no matter what the anatomy, and even what age; as long as it is the need for intervention of aortic valve disease, TAVI always can be done.

The two studies of PARTNER III and EVOLUT in 2019 are an eye-catching new research progress of TAVI technology. On this basis, the FDA and the European Drug Regulatory Agency have approved the extension of TAVI surgical indications from surgical high-risk patients with severe aortic stenosis to surgical low-risk patients, which indicates that TAVI technology will continue to develop rapidly towards the goal of the whole population in the future. It is believed that more research evidence will be published one after another, the guidelines for the diagnosis and treatment of cardiac valvular disease will change greatly, and interventional valvular technology will play a more and more important role.

5. The concept of heart team in TAVI procedure

Because of the old age of patients and high-risk factors, TAVI procedure is still relatively risky and difficult, so it is necessary to make a variety of emergency plans during the operation, including the most dangerous emergency such as heart rupture and arrest. Compared with coronary stent intervention, the probability of conversion to emergency surgery is similar, but the harm of TAVI is much higher. The risk of emergency during coronary stent was 0.2%, and the mortality rate was 1%. However, the data of 27,760 TAVI patients enrolled in 79 European centers in 2017 showed that the probability of emergency surgery was 0.76% [50]. The 3-day, perioperative, and 1-year mortality rates were 34.6%, 46%, and 78%, respectively. The average age of patients who needed emergency heart surgery was 82.4 years old, and 67.5% of the patients were female with Logistic EuroSCORE score of 17.1% and STS score of 5.8%. The analysis showed that the incidence of emergency heart surgery during TAVI decreased from 1.07% in 2013 to 0.70% in 2014 and has remained stable since then. It implies the clinical experience play important role in the procedure.

The most common causes of emergency cardiac surgery during TAVI are left ventricular perforation (28.3%) and annular rupture (21.2%) caused by guide wire. The mortality rate of patients in this situation was as high as 34.6% within 72 hours after operation. The total in-hospital mortality rate of these patients was 46.0%, and the mortality rate of patients with valvular annulus rupture was the highest (62%). The analysis also showed that the independent predictors of in-hospital death after emergency cardiac surgery were age > 85 years (OR = 1.87, P = 0.044), valvular annulus rupture (OR = 1.96, P = 0.060), and immediate emergency cardiac surgery (OR = 3.12, P = 0.037). Of these patients undergoing emergency cardiac surgery, 114 survived during hospitalization, with a 1-year survival rate of only 40.4%.

It should be emphasized that complications of TAVI are usually more critical, faster, and more difficult to predict. In particular, TAVI indication will soon be extended to low-risk patients, to ensure the safety of these patients is more important at this time. The cooperation of multiple heart teams can better ensure the safety of patients.

Perhaps the greatest contribution of TAVI technology to medical treatment is not the techniques itself or clinical effect, but a unique medical cultural phenomenon. For the first time, barriers between medical disciplines have been replaced by multidisciplinary collaboration to deal with a state of disease. As Cribier pointed out in his review of the 20th anniversary of TAVI procedure [8], the development of TAVI technology has for the first time created a model of collaboration among cardiac doctors. It is difficult for cardiologists or surgeons alone to complete all the links involved in TAVI surgery, but the two can complement each other and provide safer and effective treatment for these high-risk and elderly patients. Therefore, in many countries and regions in Europe and the United States, only TAVI cases that have been signed by the heart team can be reimbursed by the medical insurance. According to the 2012 European Society of Cardiology/European Society of Cardio-Thoracic Surgery (ESC/EACTS) guidelines for the management of cardiac valvular disease, TAVI can be considered for high-risk patients with symptomatic severe aortic valve stenosis, but requires a "heart team" comprehensive analysis and evaluation (II/B) [51]. The newly released American Heart Association/American College of Cardiology (AHA/ACC) guidelines on valvular heart disease in 2017 also give the highest level of recommendation on the importance of heart teams during TAVI procedure [52].

The American Society of Thoracic Surgeons (AATS), in conjunction with the American College of Cardiology, the Society of Cardiovascular Angiography and Intervention, and the College of Thoracic Surgeons (STS), released the latest edition of 2018 AATS/ACC/SCAI/STS Expert Consensus Systems of Care Document: Operator and Institutional Recommendations and Requirements for Transcatheter Aortic Valve Replacement [53]. The new consensus points out that in order to ensure the safety and effectiveness, TAVI procedures should be performed in centers that meet the following criteria. At least 50 TAVI cases (or 100 in 2 years) and at least 30 surgical aortic valve replacements (or 60 in 2 years) are performed in the hospital each year. The standards also include various medical quality requirements for morbidity, mortality, and quality of life within a limited time, as well as conducting quality assessment/improvement plans. The consensus also points out that TAVI operators, as members of a multidisciplinary team, should have participated in at least 100 cases of transfemoral TAVI in their career, of which at least 50 were primary operations. Surgeons on the TAVI team should have performed at least 100 surgical aortic valve replacements in their careers or at least 20 (or 50 in 2 years) in the year before the start of the TAVI program. In Chinese experts consensus about the heart team construction [44], it implies that the surgeon in TAVI team should have valve surgery experience more than 15 years and perform aortic valve surgery at least 25 cases a year. In addition, surgeons should actively participate in the TAVI procedure like wire and valve manipulation and not only just stand by.

Carl Tommaso, one of the co-chairs of the expert consensus committee, commented that the TAVI procedure safety evaluation will be used to define centers whether this operation can be performed safely or not. In the past 6 years, more and more centers have performed TAVI, and the indications are being extended to surgical low-risk elderly patients, so it is time to redefine TAVI recommendations.

Some studies have shown that there are fewer postoperative adverse events in hospitals that perform more TAVI operations, and the accumulated TAVI experience is related to the improvement of postoperative outcomes. In 2018, the *Journal of the American Medical Association Cardiology* (JAMA Cardiol) published an observational cohort study [54] that included 60,538 TAVI operations performed in 438 hospitals from 2011 to 2016, with an average age of 82.3 years. Hospitals with a high amount of surgical valve replacement (annual average ≥ 97 / year) are more likely to start TAVI in the early stage, and the amount of TAVI increases faster with time. The average TAVI cases of hospitals with high surgical valve replacement volume to those with low volume was 32 vs. 19 in the first year, 48 vs. 28 in the second year, 82 vs. 38 in the third year, and 118 vs. 54 in the fourth year ($P < 0.001$). Combined with the analysis of hospital TAVI and surgical valve replacement volume, the 30-day mortality rate in high TAVI volume hospital was lower. When the hospital also has a high volume of surgical valve replacement, the effect is more obvious. Patients with high surgical valve replacement volume and high TAVI volume had the lowest 30-day mortality (for hospitals with low surgical valve replacement volume and TAVI volume: OR = 0.77; 95%CI, 0.66–0.89). Hospitals with both high volume of surgical valve replacement and TAVI cases may have the best outcome, which confirms the importance of hospital clinic experience.

6. TAVI treatment of pure aortic valve regurgitation

The analysis of echocardiography data from Shanghai Zhongshan Hospital (including 0.3 million patients) indicates [55] that the incidence of aortic valve stenosis in China may be significantly lower than that in western countries, while aortic regurgitation (AR) is more common than aortic stenosis [56]. A retrospective data analysis from Shanghai Changhai Hospital in the past 20 years showed that the proportion of AR in patients undergoing surgical aortic valve replacement was significantly higher than that in patients with AS [57, 58]. The latest China-DVD multicenter study in 2019 showed that among the 8638 patients with valvular heart disease in China, there were 894 cases of aortic regurgitation, 430 cases of aortic stenosis, 286 cases of mitral stenosis, and 2248 cases of mitral regurgitation [59]. Patients with simple AR are still mainly treated by surgery. However, the influence of aortic regurgitation on the left ventricle and the induced symptoms of heart failure are very different from those of aortic stenosis. In patients with aortic regurgitation, the left ventricle enlarged more obviously, and the ejection fraction decreased more. But due to the late appearance of pulmonary congestion comparing with aortic stenosis, the clinical symptoms often appeared late, many patients went to see doctor very late when combined serious heart dysfunction. At this time, the patient's heart disease is not only aortic regurgitation but also left ventricular enlargement and heart failure. Even if aortic valve surgery solves valvular regurgitation, it will take longer time for heart function to recover. On the contrary, the cardiac function of many patients with aortic valve stenosis can recover in a short time after operation. Studies [60, 61] showed that about 10% AR patients are unable to undergo surgery because of old age and severe multiple organ dysfunction. Only 20% AR patients with a left ventricular ejection fraction ranging from 30% to 50% have received surgery. When the left ventricular ejection fraction is less than 30%, the proportion of patients undergoing surgery is as low as 3%. According to statistics, the annual mortality rate of patients treated with conservative medicines is as high as 10–20%, and the 10-year complication rate and mortality rate are not optimistic.

Because of the long stent structure design, the Medtronic CoreValve valve may be anchored at multiple points which may be helpful in the TAVI treatment of pure AR. In 2010, Ducrocq et al. reported that CoreValve was used to treat a high-risk AR patient with good results [62]. This is a self-expanding valve and can be implanted through the femoral artery. Its advantage lies in the long stent over 50 mm and the special three-stage fixation mechanism, in which the lower part squeezes the primary lobe through higher radial expansion, the middle part is compressed to avoid coronary artery blockage, and the upper part expands to fix to the ascending aorta and provides longitudinal coaxial stability. Therefore, even in the absence of valve calcification, the valve can theoretically be anchored in other positions. However, there are also some difficulties in the use of this valve [28, 63]. (1) Inadequate anchoring can easily lead to valve displacement, resulting in a higher incidence of secondary valve implantation and postoperative moderate and severe perivalvular leakage. Roy et al. [64] studied 43 AR patients with TAVI from 14 centers. The results showed that the rates of second valve implantation and the postoperative moderate perivalvular leakage were 19% and 21%, respectively. (2) Since the CoreValve is mainly fixed at the annulus with strong radial force, it is usually necessary to make the artificial valve diameter slightly larger than that of the autologous annulus in order to obtain sufficient radial support to make the anchoring more stable, which also leads to a higher risk of annulus tear.

Since then, the second- generation TAVI valve has higher implantation rate due to the anchoring clip design which may help to locate and fix the valve. In 2013, Seiffert et al. [65] summarized the treatment effect of JenaValve in 5five patients with pure AR without calcification. The operation was performed through apical approach, and the success rate of valve implantation was 100%. There was no obvious residual regurgitation of aortic valve, and the cardiac function of the patients recovered satisfactorily after follow-up. In 2014, a Chinese team comprised of Da et al. [66] reported the excellent results of J-Valve, the China- designed second-generation TAVI valve, in the treatment of a high-risk AR case. J-Valve is designed to be implanted through the apical approach with three U-shaped positioning keys, which can be easily self-adjusted to enter the bottom of the aortic valve sinus. After the stent valve is released, the valve can be fixed and clamped together with the positioning key to assist the radial support to anchor the valve. Since 2017 J-Valve was officially put on the market for commercial use in China. In 2019, about 800 J-Valve TAVI procedures were performed in China, in which more than half was pure AR, and the clinical effect was very satisfied. At present, the transfemoral J-Valve system has begun clinical trials in Canada and the United States with promising results [48].

In 2016 one meta-analysis [67] summarized 13 TAVI studies with 237 pure AR patients who could not tolerate surgical valve replacement. Among them, the utilization rate of self-expanding valve accounted for 79%, the implantation success rate was 77–100%, the 30-day all-cause mortality rate was 7%, and the incidence of postoperative moderate and severe valvular regurgitation was 9% (0% in JenaValve subgroup). It can be seen that although the study included JenaValve, a second-generation TAVI valve, the incidence of moderate and severe regurgitation and valve displacement after AR TAVI procedure was significantly higher than that of aortic stenosis.

In 2017 Yoon et al. [68] concluded that the new generation of TAVI valve with positioning-assisted anchoring system for the treatment of pure AR has higher implant success rate than the first-generation valve (81.1% vs. 61.3%), greatly reducing postoperative residual valvular regurgitation and perivalvular leakage (4.2% vs. 18.8%), and the probability of reimplantation of a second valve is greatly reduced (12.7% vs. 24.4%). Totally 331 AR patients underwent TAVI, with an average STS score of 6.7%. 119 cases (36%) used early valves, and 212 cases (64%) used a new generation of valvular systems. The STS score of patients with new-generation valve implantation system was lower (6.2 ± 6.7 vs. 7.6 ± 6.7), but there was no statistical difference. The new generation of valves is more likely to get through the femoral artery access (87.4% vs. 60.8%). There was no significant difference in 30-day mortality between the two groups. The 1-year all-cause mortality rates of the two groups were 24.1% and 15.6%, respectively. The 1-year all-cause mortality was related to the degree of postoperative aortic regurgitation. The mortality rate of cases with moderate and severe regurgitation was 46.1%, while mild regurgitation decreased to 21.8%. Multivariate analysis showed that more than moderate postoperative regurgitation was an independent predictor of 1-year all-cause mortality (increased by 2.85 times). And this data is not included in China's J-Valve system reports.

In 2018, De Backer et al. [69] reported 254 high-risk AR patients in 46 centers, with an average age of 74 ± 12 years, a STS score of 6.6 ± 6.2%, with first-generation valve of 43%, and second-generation valve of 57%. The success rate of new generation valve implantation was significantly higher (82% vs. 47%), valve displacement decreased (9% vs. 33%), and aortic valve regurgitation decreased (4% vs. 31%). Both small or large valve size will easily lead to valve displacement. In 2019, Takagi et al. [70] summarized the TAVI efficacy of 11 studies with 911 pure AR patients. The overall valve implantation success rate was 80.4%, of which the early valve and the new-generation valve were 67.2% and 90.2%, respectively. Moderate and severe perivalvular leakage was 7.4% (early and new-generation valves were 17.3% and 3.4%, respectively). The 30-day all-cause mortality rate was 9.5% (early and new-generation valves were 14.7% and 6.1%, respectively). During the follow-up from 4 months to 1 year, the all-cause mortality rate was 18.8% (early and new-generation valves were 32.2% and 11.8%, respectively). Vascular complications accounted for 3.9% (rates of early and new-generation valves were 6.2% and 3.0%, respectively). Life-threatening major bleeding was 5.7% (early and new-generation valves were 12.4% and 3.5%, respectively). In summary, the new generation of TAVI valve has a good therapeutic effect.

In China, there are also surgical high-risk cases in which the ascending aorta is not wide or the left ventricular outflow tract is small; some tried to use high stent self-expanding Venus A valve to treat pure AR patients. The results show that the valve displacement rate and the chance of reimplantation of the second valve are still very high (up to more than 50%). And there is also valve displacement into the ascending aorta or slipping in the left ventricle which may affect mitral valve function. These may result in doing open-chest surgery to remove the valve immediately. Therefore, this method is only suggested to be performed for high-risk patients and when other second-generation TAVI valves like J-Valve are not available.

The J-Valve valve with independent intellectual property rights in China is designed with three U-shaped positioning keys suitable for the anatomical structure of the aortic valve and sinus. The valve is released in two parts and then combined to play a role, which can more accurately locate the bottom of the aortic sinus and clamp the leaflet. J-Valve can effectively play a role in both aortic stenosis and regurgitation. A multicenter clinical study of trans-apical J-Valve in the treatment of high-risk noncalcified pure AR patients concluded data from 2014 to 2018 [71] in China. A total of 82 patients, aged 73.86.3 years, were included. The score of European cardiac surgery risk assessment system was 17.5 ± 8.1%. During the TAVI operation, four patients were converted to thoracotomy due to valve transposition, and the success rate of valve implantation was 95% (78/82). During hospitalization, one case died of moderate perivalvular leakage complicated with multiple organ failure, and one case died of pulmonary infection. There was no residual aortic regurgitation in 82.1% (64/78) patients, mild perivalvular leakage in 16.7% (13/78) patients, and permanent pacemaker placement in 7.6% (6/78) patients due to III °atrioventricular block. The left ventricular end-diastolic volume decreased from (197.7 ± 66.8) ml to (147.2 ± 53.3) ml at 1 month after TAVI. The average transvalvular gradient was (9.5 ± 4.1) mmHg, which showed good hemodynamic performance.

For the common problems of lack of calcification anchoring and aorta dilatation in AR patients, the former has been solved to a certain extent by the continuous improvement of the second-generation TAVI valve with newly designed anchoring system, while the latter is still a difficult problem that cannot be solved at present. Therefore, many patients can only choose thoracotomy or even conservative medicine treatment. In addition, compared with patients with severe AS, patients with AR are often accompanied by more serious clinical symptoms, such as pulmonary hypertension, cardiac insufficiency, and so on. At the same time, late left ventricular hypertrophy, myocardial fibrosis, and cardiac insufficiency caused by AR may not be reversed even after TAVI, so these patients tend to have a poor prognosis and need longer time of medication treatment for the heart function recovery [29]. All these problems may take physicians more efforts in clinic to get good results for those AR patients with heart dysfunction besides of the TAVI procedure.

7. Conclusion

With the continuous development of interventional valve treatment technology, the interventional treatment of aortic stenosis and aortic insufficiency is more mature; many new generations of TAVI valves are emerging, which can be more convenient for clinicians to use, which can achieve more satisfactory treatment results. As for the development of TAVI technology and the extension of follow-up time, the indications of TAVI technology are also expanding. It is reasonable to believe that TAVI technology will be the main treatment technology in the future.

Acknowledgements

I would like to thank our heart valve center of cardiac surgery department of Beijing Anzhen Hospital, Capital Medical University. Their joint efforts made our center the first unit in China to successfully carry out interventional therapy technology for all four major heart valve diseases. Thanks to president Wei Yongxiang and vice president Zhou Yujie for their consistent strong support and trust in the development of new technology in our team. Thanks to professor Meng Xu, discipline director, for his planning and design, our center began to track the latest preface technology of TAVI technology as early as 2006 and kept close academic contact with the international advanced center. Thanks for the selfless dedication and support of our center's TAVI team, including cardiac surgery, cardiology, anesthesiology, imaging, hybrid operation room, intensive care unit, ultrasound department, interventional department, etc. At the same time, I also thank TAVI teams of other heart centers in China for their support and help.

Conflict of interest

I confirm that there are no conflicts of interest.

Author details

Zhang Haibo* and Meng Xu
Cardiac Surgery Department, Beijing Anzhen Hospital, Capital Medical University, Beijing, China

*Address all correspondence to: zhanghb2318@163.com

References

[1] Stewart BF, Siscovick D, Lind BK, et al. Clinical factors associated with calcific aortic valve disease: Cardiovascular Health Study. Journal of the American College of Cardiology. 1997;**29**:630-634

[2] Otto CM, Lind BK, Kitzman DW, et al. Association of aortic valve sclerosis with cardiovascular mortality and morbidity in the elderly. The New England Journal of Medicine. 1999;**341**:142-147

[3] Nkomo VT, Gardin JM, Skelton TN, et al. Burden of valvular heart diseases: A population-based study. Lancet. 2006;**368**:1005-1011

[4] NHLBI Balloon Valvuloplasty Registry Participants. Percutaneous balloon aortic valvuloplasty. Acute and 30-day follow-up results in 674 patients from the NHLBI Balloon Valvuloplasty Registry. Circulation. 1991;**84**:2383-2397

[5] O'Neill WW. Predictors of long-term survival after percutaneous aortic valvuloplasty: Report of the Mansfield Scientific Balloon Aortic Valvuloplasty Registry. Journal of the American College of Cardiology. 1991;**17**:193-198

[6] Andersen HR, Knudsen LL, Hasenkam JM. Transluminal implantation of artificial heart valves. Description of a new expandable aortic valve and initial results with implantation by catheter technique in closed chest pigs. European Heart Journal. 1992;**13**(5):704-708

[7] Bonhoeffer P, Boudjemline Y, Saliba Z, et al. Transcatheter implantation of a bovine valve in pulmonary position: A lamb study. Circulation. 2000;**102**:813-816

[8] Cribier A. Development of transcatheter aortic valve implantation (TAVI): A 20-year odyssey. Archives of Cardiovascular Diseases. 2012;**105**(3):146-152

[9] Cribier A, Eltchaninoff H, Bash A, et al. Percutaneous transcatheter implantation of an aortic valve prosthesis for calcific aortic stenosis first human case description. Circulation. 2002;**106**(24):3006-3008

[10] Webb JG, Chandavimol M, Thompson CR, et al. Percutaneous aortic valve implantation retrograde from the femoral artery. Circulation. 2006;**113**:842-850

[11] Lichtenstein SV, Cheung A, Ye J, et al. Transapical transcatheter aortic valve implantation in humans: Initial clinical experience. Circulation. 2006;**114**:591-596

[12] Walther T, Simon P, Dewey T, et al. Transapical minimally invasive aortic valve implantation: Multicenter experience. Circulation. 2007;**116**:I240-I245

[13] Grube E, Laborde JC, Zickmann B, et al. First report on a human percutaneous transluminal implantation of a self-expanding valve prosthesis for interventional treatment of aortic valve stenosis. Catheterization and Cardiovascular Interventions. 2005;**66**:465-469

[14] Vahanian A, Alfieri O, Andreotti F, et al. Guidelines on the management of valvular heart disease (version 2012) The Joint Task Force on the Management of Valvular Heart Disease of the European Society of Cardiology (ESC) and the European Association for Cardio-Thoracic Surgery (EACTS). European Heart Journal. 2013;**66**(2):E1-E42

[15] Leon MB, Smith CR, Mack M, et al. Transcatheter aortic-valve implantation

for aortic stenosis in patients who cannot undergo surgery. The New England Journal of Medicine. 2010;**363**(17):1597-1607

[16] Leon MB, Smith CR, Mack MJ, et al. Transcatheter or surgical aortic-valve replacement in intermediate-risk patients. The New England Journal of Medicine. 2016;**374**(17):1609-1620

[17] Popma JJ, Deeb GM, Yakubov SJ, et al. Transcatheter aortic-valve replacement with a self-expanding valve in low-risk patients. The New England Journal of Medicine. 2019;**380**(18):1706-1715

[18] Mack MJ, Leon MB, Thourani VH, et al. Transcatheter aortic valve replacement with a balloon-expandable valve in low-risk patients. The New England Journal of Medicine. 2019;**380**(18):1695-1705

[19] Durko AP, Osnabrugge RL, Van Mieghem NM, et al. Annual number of candidates for transcatheter aortic valve implantation per country: Current estimates and future projections. European Heart Journal. 2018;**39**(28):2635-2642

[20] Iung B, Delgado V, Rosenhek R, et al. Contemporary presentation and management of valvular heart disease in Europe: The EURObservational Research Programme Valvular Heart Disease II Registry. Circulation. 2019;**140**:1156-1169

[21] Sawaya FJ, Spaziano M, Lefevre T, et al. Comparison between the SAPIEN S3 and the SAPIEN XT transcatheter heart valves: A single-center experience. World Journal of Cardiology. 2016;**8**(12):735-745

[22] Tchétché D, Windecker S, Kasel AM, et al. 1-year outcomes of the centera-eu trial assessing a novel self-expanding transcatheter heart valve. JACC. Cardiovascular Interventions. 2019;**12**(7):673-680

[23] Schulz E, Jabs A, Gori T, et al. Transcatheter aortic valve implantation with the new-generation Evolut R: Comparison with CoreValve(R) in a single center cohort. IJC Heart & Vasculature. 2016;**12**:52-56

[24] Noble S, Stortecky S, Heg D, et al. Comparison of procedural and clinical outcomes with Evolut R versus Medtronic CoreValve: A Swiss TAVI registry analysis. EuroIntervention. 2017;**12**(18):e2170-e2176

[25] Gomes B, Geis NA, Chorianopoulos E, et al. Improvements of procedural results with a new-generation self-expanding transfemoral aortic valve prosthesis in comparison to the old generation device. Journal of Interventional Cardiology. 2017;**30**(1):72-78

[26] Asch FM, Vannan MA, Singh S, et al. Hemodynamic and echocardiographic comparison of the Lotus and CoreValve transcatheter aortic valves in patients with high and extreme surgical risk: An analysis from the REPRISE III randomized controlled trial. Circulation. 2018;**137**(24):2557-2567

[27] Lanz J, Kim WK, Walther T, et al. Safety and efficacy of a self-expanding versus a balloon-expandable bioprosthesis for transcatheter aortic valve replacement in patients with symptomatic severe aortic stenosis: A randomised non-inferiority trial. Lancet. 2019;**394**(10209):1619-1628

[28] Seiffert M, Bader R, Kappert U, et al. Initial German experience with transapical implantation of a second-generation transcatheter heart valve for

the treatment of aortic regurgitation. JACC. Cardiovascular Interventions. 2014;**7**(10):1168-1174

[29] Schlingloff F, Schafer U, Frerker C, et al. Transcatheter aortic valve implantation of a second-generation valve for pure aortic regurgitation: Procedural outcome, haemodynamic data and follow-up. Interactive Cardiovascular and Thoracic Surgery. 2014;**19**(3):388-393

[30] Zhu D, Chen W, Peng L, et al. Valve sizing for pure aortic regurgitation during transcatheter aortic valve replacement: Deformation dynamic of the aortic annulus in different valve pathology may be different. JACC. Cardiovascular Interventions. 2015;**8**(2):372-373

[31] Holzhey D, Linke A, Treede H, et al. Intermediate follow-up results from the multicenter engager European pivotal trial. The Annals of Thoracic Surgery. 2013;**96**(6):2095-2100

[32] Gao R. Current situation of heart valvular disease in China. Huaxi Medicine. 2018;**33**(2):127-131

[33] Liu FZ, Xue YM, Liao HT, et al. Five-year epidemiological survey of valvular heart disease: Changes in morbidity, etiological spectrum and management in a cardiovascular center of Southern China. Journal of Thoracic Disease. 2014;**6**(12):1724-1730

[34] Yifan B. 20 years changes of surgical treatment risk factors for adult heart valvular disease [thesis]. Shanghai: Doctoral Dissertation of Second Military Medical University; 2012

[35] Xiang C. Analysis of risk factors of death in hospital after adult aortic valve replacement [thesis]. Shanghai: Doctoral Dissertation of Second Military Medical University; 2012

[36] Junbo GE, Daxin Z, Pan W, et al. A case of percutaneous aortic valve implantation and the main points of operation. Chinese Journal of Interventional Cardiology. 2010;**18**(5):243-246

[37] Structural Cardiology Committee of Chinese College of Cardiovascular Physicians. Chinese experts consensus on transcatheter aortic valve replacement. Chinese Journal of Interventional Cardiology. 2015;**23**(12):661-667

[38] Otto CM, Kumbhani DJ, Alexander KP, et al. 2017 ACC expert consensus decision pathway for transcatheter aortic valve replacement in the management of adults with aortic stenosis. Journal of the American College of Cardiology. 2017;**69**(10):1313-1346

[39] Structural Cardiology Committee of Chinese College of Cardiovascular Physicians, Chinese Society of Cardiology. Chinese experts consensus of team construction and operation standard on transcatheter aortic valve replacement. Chinese Journal of Interventional Cardiology. 2018;**26**(1):2-6

[40] Wu Y et al. Experts consensus on clinical pathway of transcatheter aortic valve replacement in China. Chinese Circulation Journal. 2018;**33**(12):22-29

[41] Group of Echocardiography, Chinese Medical Association. Expert consensus on perioperative echocardiographic examination of transcatheter aortic valve implantation. Chinese Journal of Ultrasonography. 2018;**27**(2):93-107

[42] Cardiovascular Anesthesia Branch of Chinese Society of Cardiothoracic and Vascular Anesthesiology. Anesthesia experts consensus on

clinical pathway management in TAVR surgery. Journal of Clinical Anesthesia. 2018;**34**(11):1118-1124

[43] Chunsheng W, Lai W, Xu M, et al. Committee of Minimally Invasive Cardiovascular Surgery, National Experts Committee on Cardiovascular Diseases. China multidisciplinary expert consensus on transcatheter aortic valve implantation. Chinese Journal of Thoracic and Cardiovascular Surgery. 2018;**34**(12):705-712

[44] Xu M, Xu Z, Haibo Z, et al. Chinese expert consensus on transcatheter aortic valve implantation heart team construction and cardiac surgeon responsibility. Chinese Journal of Thoracic and Cardiovascular Surgery. 2019;**35**(12):717-720

[45] Haibo Z, Xu M, Wang S, et al. Transcatheter mitral valve in valve technique treatment with domestic J valve system. Chinese Journal of Thoracic and Cardiovascular Surgery. 2019;**35**(6):331-333

[46] Feng Y, Zhao ZG, Baccaro J, et al. First-in-man implantation of a pre-packaged self-expandable dry-tissue transcatheter aortic valve. European Heart Journal. 2018;**39**(8):713

[47] Zhu D, Wei L, Cheung A, et al. Treatment of pure aortic regurgitation using a second-generation transcatheter aortic valve implantation system. Journal of the American College of Cardiology. 2016;**67**(23):2803-2805

[48] Hensey M, Murdoch DJ, Sathananthan J, et al. First-in-human experience of a new-generation transfemoral transcatheter aortic valve for the treatment of severe aortic regurgitation: The J-valve transfemoral system. EuroIntervention. 2019;**14**(15):e1553-e1555

[49] Bevan GH, Zidar DA, Josephson RA, et al. Mortality due to aortic stenosis in the United States, 2008-2017. JAMA. 2019;**321**(22):2236-2238

[50] Eggebrecht H, Vaquerizo B, Moris C, et al. Incidence and outcomes of emergent cardiac surgery during transfemoral transcatheter aortic valve implantation (TAVI): insights from the European Registry on Emergent Cardiac Surgery during TAVI (EuRECS-TAVI). European Heart Journal. 2017;**39**(8):676-684

[51] Joint Task Force on the Management of Valvular Heart Disease of the European Society of Cardiology (ESC), European Association for Cardio-Thoracic Surgery (EACTS), Vahanian A, et al. Guidelines on the management of valvular heart disease (version 2012). European Heart Journal. 2012;**33**(19):2451-2496

[52] Nishimura RA, Otto CM, Bonow RO, et al. AHA/ACC guideline for the management of patients with valvular heart disease: A report of the American College of Cardiology/American Heart Association Task Force on Practice Guidelines. Journal of the American College of Cardiology. 2014;**63**(22):e57-e185

[53] Bavaria JE, Tommaso CL, Brindis RG, et al. 2018 AATS/ACC/SCAI/STS expert consensus Systems of Care Document: Operator and institutional recommendations and requirements for Transcatheter aortic valve replacement. The Journal of Thoracic and Cardiovascular Surgery. 2018;**73**(3):340-374

[54] Mao J, Rita FR, John DC, et al. Association between hospital surgical aortic valve replacement volume and transcatheter aortic valve replacement outcomes. JAMA Cardiology. 2018;**3**(11):1070-1078

[55] Pan W, Zhou D, Cheng L, et al. Candidates for transcatheter aortic valve implantation may be fewer in China. International Journal of Cardiology. 2013;**168**:e133-e134

[56] Pan W, Zhou D, Cheng L, et al. Aortic regurgitation is more prevalent than aortic stenosis in Chinese elderly population: Implications for transcatheter aortic valve replacement. International Journal of Cardiology. 2015;**201**:547-548

[57] Yifan B. 20 years risk factors changes of adult heart valvular disease surgical treatment [Doctoral dissertation]. Shanghai, China: Shanghai Second Military Medical University; 2012. p. 4

[58] Xiang C. Risk factors analysis of death in hospital after adult aortic valve replacement [Doctoral dissertation]. Shanghai, China: Shanghai Second Military Medical University; 2012. p. 5

[59] Xiling Q, Xu H, Qingrong L, et al. Analysis of diagnosis and treatment of senile degenerative heart valvular disease in China. Chinese Circulation Journal. 2019;**34**(8):771-776

[60] Iung B, Baron G, Butchart EG, et al. A prospective survey of patients with valvular heart disease in Europe: The euro heart survey on valvular heart disease. European Heart Journal. 2003;**24**(13):1231-1243

[61] Dujardin KS, Enriquez-Sarano M, Schaff HV, et al. Mortality and morbidity of aortic regurgitation in clinical practice. A long-term follow-up study. Circulation. 1999;**99**(14):1851-1857

[62] Ducrocq G, Himbert D, Hvass U, et al. Compassionate aortic valve implantation for severe aortic regurgitation. The Journal of Thoracic and Cardiovascular Surgery. 2010;**140**(4):930-932

[63] Wei L, Liu H, Zhu L, et al. A new transcatheter aortic valve replacement system for predominant aortic regurgitation implantation of the J-valve and early outcome. JACC. Cardiovascular Interventions. 2015;**8**(14):1831-1841

[64] Roy DA, Schaefer U, Guetta V, et al. Transcatheter aortic valve implantation for pure severe native aortic valve regurgitation. Journal of the American College of Cardiology. 2013;**61**(15):1577-1584

[65] Seiffert M, Diemert P, Koschyk D, et al. Transapical implantation of a second-generation transcatheter heart valve in patients with noncalcified aortic regurgitation. JACC. Cardiovascular Interventions. 2013;**6**(6):590-597

[66] Zhu D, Hu J, Meng W, et al. Successful transcatheter aortic valve implantation for pure aortic regurgitation using a new second generation self-expanding J-ValveTM system—The first in-man implantation. Heart, Lung & Circulation. 2015;**24**(4):411-414

[67] Franzone A, Piccolo R, Siontis GCM, et al. Transcatheter aortic valve replacement for the treatment of pure native aortic valve regurgitation a systematic review. JACC: Cardiovascular Interventions. 2016;**9**(22):2308-2317

[68] Yoon S-H, Schmidt T, Bleiziffer S, et al. Transcatheter aortic valve replacement in pure native aortic valve regurgitation. Journal of the American College of Cardiology. 2017;**70**(22):2752-2763

[69] De Backer O, Pilgrim T, Simonato M, et al. Usefulness of transcatheter aortic valve implantation for treatment of pure native aortic valve regurgitation.

The American Journal of Cardiology. 2018;**122**(6):1028-1035

[70] Takagi H, Hari Y, Kawai N, et al. Meta-analysis and meta-regression of transcatheter aortic valve implantation for pure native aortic regurgitation. Heart, Lung & Circulation. 2019;**29**(5):729-741

[71] Luo Y, Lulu L, Jun S, et al. Early clinical results of transcatheter aortic valve replacement with J-valve for high risk pure aortic regurgitation. Chinese Journal of Thoracic and Cardiovascular Surgery. 2019;**26**(8):737743

Section 2

Fontan Therapies

Chapter 6

Physiopathological Approach of the Fontan Patient for Noncardiac Surgery for the Anesthesiologist

Yamile Muñoz, María José Sáenz and Renzo Cifuentes

Abstract

Since 1971, when Dr. Francis Fontan and collaborators described a surgical technique that restored pulmonary flow in patients with tricuspid atresia and despite the fact that it has had modifications over time, the impact on the survival of these patients has been notable. It is currently known as the Fontan procedure and is indicated to treat single ventricle congenital heart defects. Thanks to the great advances in the field of congenital heart surgery, as well as better pediatric cardiology and intensive care management, the survival of patients with congenital heart defects has increased significantly, among whom are patients with univentricular or single ventricle physiology. The objective of this chapter is to provide the anesthesiologist with useful and applicable concepts in the evaluation and perioperative management of patients with a Fontan repair, especially for noncardiac surgeries.

Keywords: congenital heart disease (CHD), chronic heart failure (CHF), single ventricle (SV), Fontan procedure, Fontan physiology, Fontan failure, pulmonary vascular resistance (PVR), systemic vascular resistance (SVR), total cavopulmonary connection (TCPC), cardiac output (CO), cardiac index (CI), preoperative evaluation, intraoperative management

1. Introduction

Univentricular patients in the stage of Fontan palliation have a higher perioperative risk than their counterparts with normal hearts.

The diagnosis and treatment of children with congenital heart disease (CHD) has improved significantly over the last decades. The incidence of CHD has remained stable; the natural history of the lesions and overall survival rate have also changed notably. Advances made in surgical procedures and techniques, in concert with improvements in diagnosis, anesthesia practices, intensive care, and medical treatments, have transformed many of these fatal lesions into manageable chronic conditions [1].

Many more of these patients are surviving with this physiology than could have been contemplated 30 years ago and nowadays they seek medical attention for other causes different from their cardiovascular conditions that require surgical noncardiac procedures.

A normal biventricular cardiovascular system consists of a double circuit, pulmonary and systemic, connected in series and powered by a double pump. Many complex cardiac malformations are characterized by the existence of only one functional ventricle. This single ventricle (SV) has to maintain both the systemic and the pulmonary circulations, which at birth are not connected in series but in parallel [2].

Regardless of the exact nature of the connections, the completed circulation is often described as one having a single energy source, the systemic ventricle [3].

The survival improvement of patients with univentricular physiology is due to the development of the staged palliation approach for complex congenital heart lesions not suitable for biventricular repair. The final Fontan stage results in the conversion of a parallel circulation, to a pulmonary and systemic circulation that is in series regardless of the underlying cardiac anatomy [2, 4]. Such lesions include hypoplastic left-heart syndrome (HLHS), tricuspid atresia, unbalanced atrioventricular septal defects, double-inlet left ventricle, double-outlet right ventricle, and some forms of heterotaxy syndrome [5].

The objective of this chapter is to provide anesthesiologists the conceptual aspects applicable to the preoperative evaluation and perioperative management of patients with the unique Fontan physiology.

2. The Fontan patient

2.1 Staged palliation

First stage: The goals of initial palliation are to provide unobstructed systemic blood flow, well-balanced pulmonary and systemic circulations with controlled pulmonary blood flow, and unobstructed pulmonary and systemic venous return (including unrestricted atrial level mixing of venous returns). The elevated pulmonary vascular resistance (PVR) characteristic of the newborn period requires a staged approach to achieve these long-term goals that include normalization of the ventricular volume load and provision of normal systemic oxygen delivery. The success of a shunt is evaluated based on the relief of cyanosis, without a significant volume overload of the ventricle, and the induction of pulmonary growth without causing major changes to PVR. The systemic to pulmonary shunt is designed to last 4–6 months, sufficient time for the PVR to drop, allowing a partial cavopulmonary connection to be created safely (**Figure 1**).

Second stage: The superior cavopulmonary connection (SCPC, bidirectional Glenn or hemi-Fontan) is the surgical anastomosis of the superior vena cava (SVC) to the pulmonary artery (PA) and has a significant benefit on cardiac function. The second-stage procedure diminish the volume load on the SV while maintaining systemic oxygen delivery. Therefore, the ventricular work-load approximates that of the systemic ventricle in a biventricular circulation. One of the critical features of the second-stage procedure is the opportunity for the ventricle to have enough time for remodeling following the removal of the volume load prior to Fontan completion (**Figure 2**). In addition, this stage provides the opportunity to address other anatomic and physiologic abnormalities (including atrioventricular valve regurgitation, PA distortion) in the same surgery, optimizing the chances of a successful Fontan completion later on [4].

Third stage: In 1971, Francis Fontan and colleagues described a surgical technique for successful palliation of patients with tricuspid atresia [3]. Subsequently, this technique has been applied to treat most forms of functional SV. Typically, 1–3 years after the second stage, the inferior vena cava (IVC) is connected surgically to the PA to complete the Fontan procedure [5].

There are three different types of Fontan palliation:

- The atriopulmonary connection (APC) consists of the right atrium connected directly to the PA. Although this surgical reconstruction is not performed

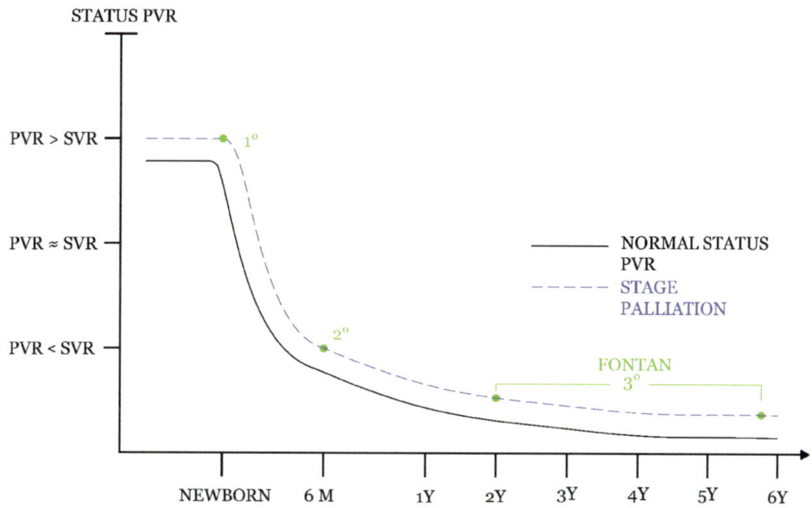

Figure 1.
Changes in PVR according to time and the appropriate age for performing stage palliation until completing the Fontan procedure for complex congenital heart disease that does not qualify for biventricular repair (PVR, pulmonary vascular resistance; SVR, systemic vascular resistance).

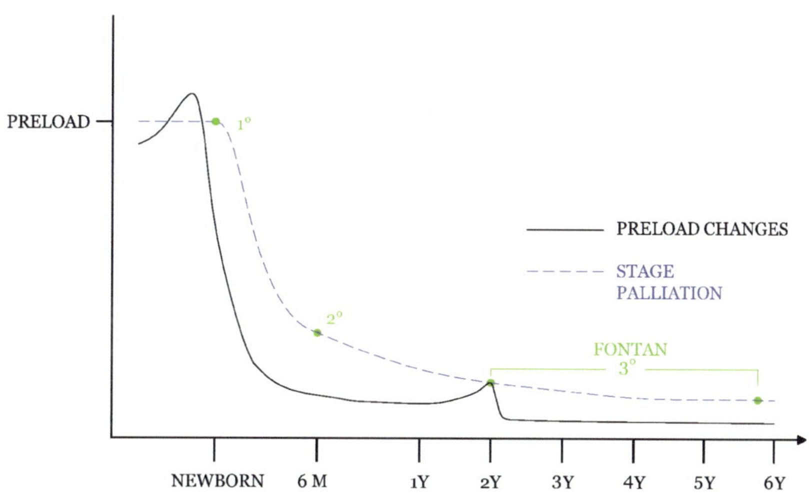

Figure 2.
Changes in the preload according to time and the appropriate age for performing stage palliation until completing the Fontan procedure for complex congenital heart disease that does not qualify for biventricular repair.

in modern practice, patients with APCs are presenting to the perioperative setting as adults. The Fontan procedure has been considerably modified since the description of a direct APC by Fontan. Several modifications were subsequently proposed in an effort to improve hemodynamic function and counteract progressive atrial dilation [6].

- The intracardiac total cavopulmonary connection, or lateral tunnel, consists of a SVC surgically connected directly to the right PA. IVC traverses through the atrium via a baffle directly to the PA.

- The extracardiac cavopulmonary connection also consists of a direct anastomosis of the SVC to the PA. However, an extracardiac conduit is used to route IVC blood directly to the PA without traversing the right atrium [5, 7].

Initially, adult survivors were mainly APC Fontan patients, but increasing numbers of both forms of TCPC Fontan patients now survive to adult life [7]. The extracardiac cavopulmonary connection is the main method employed currently in surgical centers.

2.2 Fontan anatomy

The systemic venous blood passively entering the pulmonary circulation through a total cavopulmonary anastomosis (TCPA). Blood bypasses the right atrium via a baffle or a conduit. Blood is oxygenated in the lungs and enters the pulmonary venous system reaching the left atrium. The right and left atrium now function as a common pulmonary venous atrium (CPVA). A single functional ventricle actively drives blood flow through the systemic arteries and capillaries, with systemic venous return passively entering the pulmonary circulation. The final Fontan stage results in the conversion of a parallel circulation to a pulmonary and systemic circulation that is in series [2, 5] (**Figure 3**).

2.3 Fontan physiology

By creating a TCPC, a new portal system is made. A portal system occurs when one capillary bed pools blood into another capillary bed through veins without passing through the heart.

The Fontan morphophysiology has two essential components. First, the presence of a SV pumping oxygenated blood to the systemic circulation, this ventricle can be either, a morphologic right or left depending on the type of CHD. The second

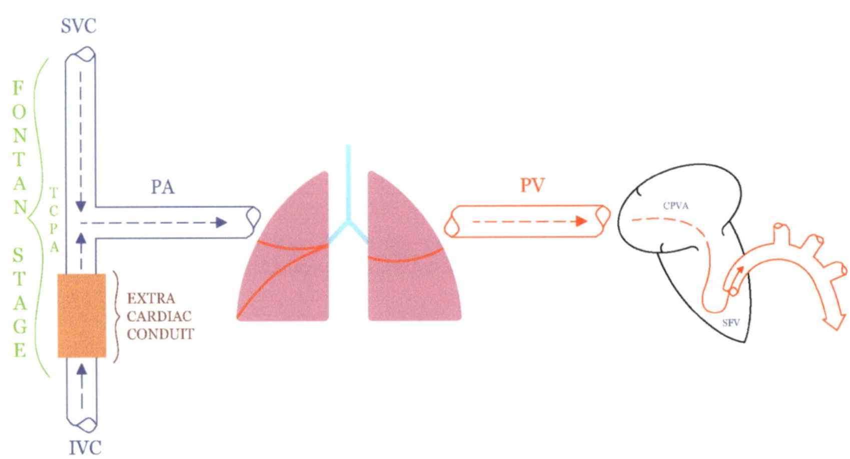

Figure 3.
Fontan anatomy. Shows how systemic venous blood passively enters the pulmonary artery (PA) circulation through a total cavopulmonary anastomosis (TCPA). Blood prevents the right atrium through a baffle or conduit. Blood is oxygenated in the lungs and enters the pulmonary venous (PV) system reaching the left atrium. The right and left atrium now function as a common pulmonary venous atrium (CPVA). A single functional ventricle (SFV) actively drives blood flow through the systemic arteries and capillaries, with a systemic venous return that passively enters the pulmonary circulation. The final stage of Fontan results in the conversion of a parallel circulation to a pulmonary and systemic circulation that is in series.

component is that the systemic venous return will reach the pulmonary arterial system without direct influence of a pumping chamber [2, 5].

The driving force that maintains adequate blood flow and therefore cardiac output (CO), is the pressure difference between the central venous pressure (CVP) and the common atrial pressure (CAP), that is also known as the transpulmonary gradient, for it to be adequate requires a well-functioning SV, decrease afterload and sufficient preload [5] (**Figure 4**).

The Fontan operation produces a state of chronic low CO [8] and relies on nonpulsatile, passive flow of caval blood to the PAs. Because there is not a sub-pulmonary ventricle, the circulation relies on low pulmonary pressures and low PVR. Forward flow through the pulmonary vasculature depends on a differential between the CVP and CAP [5]. Systemic venous hypertension is necessary to drive blood flow through the pulmonary vasculature with systemic venous pressure typically 5 mmHg higher than the pulmonary venous-atrial pressure [7].

2.4 Fenestration

An important feature of Fontan procedures, particularly lateral tunnel TCPC, is the fenestration or a surgically created small opening between the Fontan baffle pathway and the atrium. This 4-mm hole serves as a "pop-off" during times of high PVR and in essence maintains CO at the expense of a right-to-left shunt [5, 9] (**Figure 4**).

There is evidence including a prospective randomized trial that fenestration decreases the incidence of prolonged post-operative effusions, reduce post-operative lengths of hospital stay, and lessen the need for early reinterventions [4].

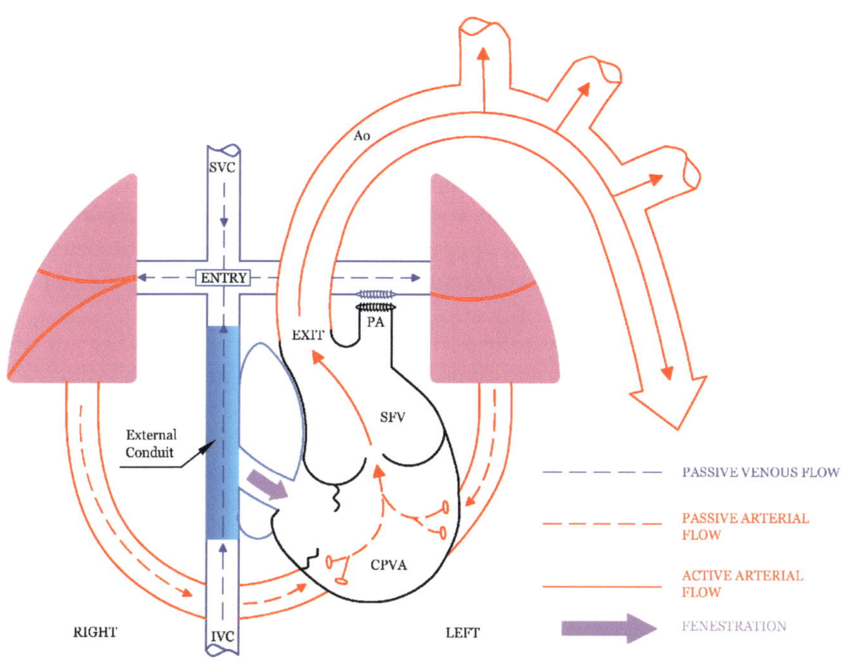

Figure 4.
Fontan physiology. The right-to-left shunt through the fenestration allows the systemic venous blood to bypass the Fontan portal system, thereby increasing the single ventricle preload, increasing cardiac output, and decreasing systemic venous congestion at expense of cyanosis that results from a lower arterial oxygen saturation (SVC, superior vena cava; IVC, inferior vena cava; Ao, aorta; PA, pulmonary artery; SFV, single functional ventricle; CPVA, common pulmonary venous atrium).

The right-to-left shunt through the fenestration allows the systemic venous blood to bypass the Fontan portal system, thereby increasing the SV preload, increasing CO, and decreasing systemic venous congestion at expense of cyanosis that results from a lower arterial oxygen saturation [9, 10].

Theoretically, the fenestration poses a risk for systemic embolic events and persistent cyanosis; however, the improved CO may have beneficial effects on oxygen delivery and will also help to alleviate the congestion felt in upstream organs, particularly the liver [2, 5].

2.5 Fontan failure

Though life-saving, the univentricular Fontan circulation does not reproduce biventricular physiology and although generally well tolerated in childhood, it seems to be less well tolerated over time, affecting organ systems outside the heart. Fontan physiology can best be thought of as a man-made form of chronic heart failure (CHF) [10] and there are a significant number of medical complications associated with the long-term. There is evidence that circulatory failure rather than ventricular failure is most important in the failing Fontan.

Griffiths et al. evaluated the outcomes of failing Fontan patients listed for transplant and observed decreased survival in patients with preserved ventricular function compared with those with impaired ventricular function [11]. The clinical deterioration can occur in the absence of ventricular dysfunction, suggesting that distinct mechanisms are contributive in comparison with heart failure patients from other etiologies.

Depiction of the hemodynamic profile of Fontan failure has been similar to traditional heart failure: elevated CVP, pulmonary capillary wedge pressure and systemic vascular resistance (SVR) with a low cardiac index (CI). Hebson et al. [12] evaluated the hemodynamic profile of a symptomatic adult Fontan (SAF) cohort with significant symptoms such as refractory edema, ascites, protein-losing enteropathy (PLE) or considerable exercise intolerance regardless of ventricular function. In the SAF patients, although CVP and pulmonary capillary wedge pressures were elevated, SVR index was low and CI was preserved even in the context of more severe symptoms. This suggests additional mechanisms influencing the hemodynamics and contributing to the symptoms of Fontan failure.

Fontan patients cannot proportionately augment their CO above a certain threshold, thus potentiating renal hypoperfusion and leading to refractory symptoms [12] and in cases where the systemic ventricle functions poorly, the heart can make an already compromised circulation worse.

In a biventricular system, systolic performance will only affect CO at rest when the ventricular function is severely depressed. In a normal subject, CO is not influenced by an increase of PVR up to 5 Woods Units. In Fontan patients, PVR is the primary modulator of CO. Failing Fontans typically have a high PVR. The loss of pulsatile flow after TCPC affects the usual vasoreactivity of the pulmonary bed. Ideally the lung vessels should be slightly oversized with low resistance. However, more frequently the abnormal development may result in relative hypoplasia of the large vessels coupled with endothelial dysfunction.

In all Fontan patients, an increase in PVR is invariably associated with a decrease in CO. If PVR is low, a reasonable output is achieved in patients with normal or moderately depressed ventricular function. However, severely depressed ventricular function results in low output [2] (**Figure 5**).

Late Fontan failure might present gradually and insidiously over years. The nature of Fontan failure is heterogenous, it is likely that not all patients "fail" in the same way, and each patient should be evaluated individually when looking for underlying causes [12].

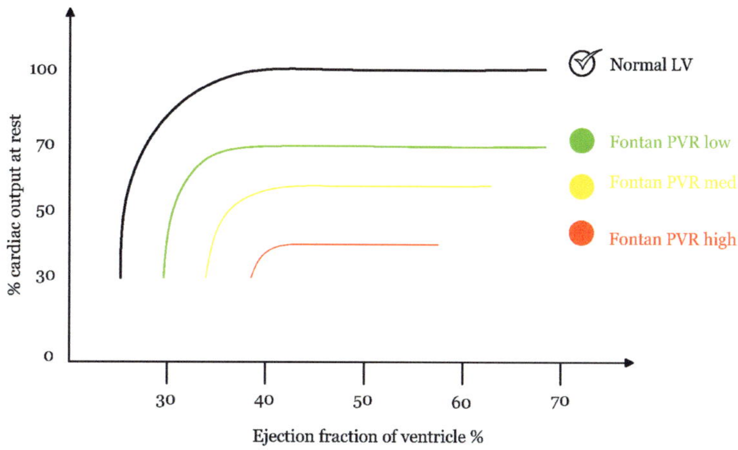

Figure 5.
Modulation of CO by PVR in normal and Fontan patients. In Fontan patients, PVR is the primary modulator of CO. If PVR is low, a reasonable CO is achieved in patients with normal or moderately depressed ventricular function. However, severely depressed ventricular function results in low CO (CO, cardiac output; PVR, pulmonary vascular resistance; LV, left ventricle).

The circulatory problem in Fontan is the limit in the preload created primarily by the damming effect of this neoportal system. The strategy is to maximize the efficiency of this system, which could have better outcomes than more traditional heart failure therapies [2].

The components that make up the Fontan system are critically important in the overall function of the Fontan circuit. These components include the venoarterial Fontan connection itself, PAs, pulmonary capillary network, pulmonary veins, and the venoatrial connection. Impairment at any level of this portal system will have profound consequences on the output of the Fontan circuit [2] (**Figure 6**). Impairments at any component level include, but are not limited to, stenosis, hypoplasia, distortion, vasoconstriction, pulmonary vascular disease, loss or exclusion

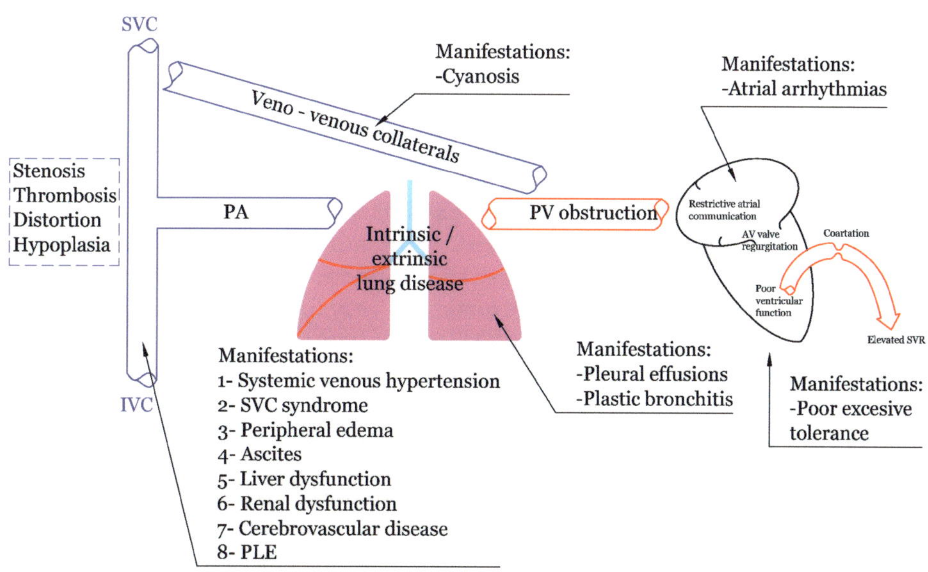

Figure 6.
The failing Fontan (PA, pulmonary artery; PV, pulmonary vein; AV, atrioventricular; SVR, systemic vascular resistance; SVC, superior vena cava; IVC, inferior vena cava; PLE, protein-losing enteropathy).

of large vessels or microvessels, turbulence and flow collision, flow mismatch and obstruction by external compression [2].

Bypassing the pulmonary vasculature can partially reverse the restrictions to CO imposed by the neoportal system. A Fontan fenestration allows flow to bypass the neoportal system, which results in venous decongestion and increase in CO.

However, while a fenestration can increase overall output, it does so at the expense of diminished arterial oxygen saturation. Nevertheless, in the setting of a fenestration, the increase in CO can result in an increase in peripheral oxygen delivery even if the saturation is diminished.

The strategy to manage a failing Fontan starts by determining modifiable conditions and intervene if it is deem necessary. The first step is imaging, using transthoracic echocardiography (TTE) and cardiac magnetic resonance (CMR) to obtain a full image of the Fontan anatomy. Assessment of atrioventricular valve regurgitation could be difficult therefore the use of transesophageal echocardiography (TEE) is needed sometimes. Catheter-based intervention is used if obstruction is identified. Surgical interventions are necessary in certain cases.

The goal of the management of the patient with Fontan physiology is to preserve symptom-free survival for as long as possible.

3. Preoperative evaluation of the Fontan patient

3.1 Perioperative risk stratification

Anesthesiologists outside of referral pediatric cardiovascular hospitals should be familiar with the anatomy, physiology, long-term manifestations and unique perioperative management of patients with Fontan palliation, and in the preoperative anesthesia consultation it is of paramount importance to define if this group of patients have an increased perioperative risk.

Faraoni et al. investigated the post-operative outcomes in children with and without CHD undergoing noncardiac surgery [1]. This study was performed using data from the 2012 pediatric database of the American College of Surgeons National Surgical Quality Improvement Program (ACS NSQIP Pediatric). They included elective versus emergent surgery, and different surgical types (i.e., thoracic, neurological, orthopedic, general pediatric (including ear, nose, and throat), plastics and urogynecology).

Children with CHD were classified into three groups: minor, major and severe CHD, as defined in the ACS NSQIP database, based on residual lesion burden and cardiovascular functional status (**Table 1**).

This authors evaluated in the cohort of patients if the presence of major or severe CHD is associated with an increased risk of anesthesia and surgery. Of the 51,008 children included in the database, 4520 children with CHD underwent noncardiac surgery. After propensity score matching, they included 2805 children with minor CHD, 1272 with major CHD, and 417 with severe CHD. The overall mortality was significantly higher in children presenting moderate (3.9%) and severe (8.2%) CHD compared with controls (1.2% and 1.7% respectively). No statistical difference was observed in children with minor CHD (1.5%) and their controls (1%).

The conclusions of the authors are children with major and severe CHD undergoing noncardiac surgery have an increased risk of mortality, and a higher incidence of post-operative reintubation compared with matched controls undergoing comparable procedures. In the study, overall mortality in children with CHD was 2.8% compared with 1.2% in children without CHD, corresponding to a 2.3-fold higher mortality rate in children with CHD. In conclusion, children with major or

Minor CHD:
• Cardiac condition with or without medication and maintenance (e.g., atrial septal defect, small-to-moderate ventricular septal defect with no symptoms) • Repair of congenital heart defect with normal cardiovascular function and no medication
Major CHD:
• Repair of congenital heart defect with residual hemodynamic abnormality with or without medications (e.g., Tetralogy of Fallot with wide open pulmonary insufficiency, HLHS including stage 1 repair)
Severe CHD:
• Uncorrected cyanotic heart disease • Patients with any documented pulmonary hypertension • Patients with ventricular dysfunction requiring medication • Listed for heart transplant
CHD, congenital heart disease; HLHS, hypoplastic left-heart syndrome.

Table 1.
Groups of children with CHD.

severe CHD who undergo noncardiac surgery have an increased risk of mortality with a higher incidence of life-threatening postoperative outcomes compared with children without CHD [1].

Then Faraoni et al., developed a validation of a risk stratification score for children with CHD undergoing noncardiac surgery [13]. The objective of this study was to identify the predictors for in-hospital mortality, and to develop a risk stratification score that could be used to help decision making and the development of perioperative management guidelines. This study was performed using data from the 2012, 2013, and 2014 pediatric databases of the ACS NSQIP and included all children with major or severe CHD as previously defined. They were able to identify eight predictors for in-hospital mortality in children with major and severe CHD undergoing noncardiac surgery: four were preoperative markers of critical illness (inotropic support, mechanical ventilation, preoperative cardiopulmonary resuscitation (CPR) and acute or chronic kidney injury), the type of lesion (e.g., single ventricle physiology (SVP)) and the functional severity of heart disease (e.g., severe CHD). All of them were excellent predictors of in-hospital mortality (**Table 2**).

Children with SVP were identified to be at high risk for perioperative complications and at increased risk of in-hospital mortality regardless of their functional status. Although ACS NSQIP Pediatric database allows identification of patients with SVP, does not provide accurate information on their specific stage of palliation [13].

The 2018 ACC/AHA guidelines for the management of adults with CHD (ACHD) stated that patients with ACHD may have greater operative risk than patients without ACHD. The guidelines recommend optimization before and close surveillance after invasive procedures regardless of the complexity of the anatomic defect or type of procedure. In patients with ACHD, especially those with complex disease (ACHD AP classification II and III) and/or whose disease has progressed (stages B, C, D), noncardiac surgical and interventional procedures should be performed in a hospital with or in consultation with experts in ACHD when possible. Because the inability to access resources or urgent conditions may preclude transfer or timely consultation, collaboration with members of the multidisciplinary ACHD team may be helpful [14].

1. Critical illness: inotropic support, mechanical ventilation, preoperative CPR, acute or chronic kidney injury
2. SVP
3. Functional severity: major CHD and severe CHD
CPR, cardiopulmonary resuscitation; SVP, single ventricle physiology; CHD, congenital heart disease.

Table 2.
Predictors of in-hospital mortality.

3.2 Multisystem approach for Fontan patient evaluation

Even though mortality in patients with SVP who undergo staged palliation has decreased significantly over the past decades, Fontan physiology and its long-term complications (e.g., arrhythmias, circulatory failure, multi-organic compromise, etc.) continue to pose significant challenges in the management of children and adults requiring anesthesia for noncardiac surgical or invasive procedures.

The preoperative evaluation of the patient with Fontan physiology involves a thorough history and physical examination as well as review of recent cardiovascular imaging studies, using a multisystem approach with attention to the unique characteristics of this patient population (**Figure 7**).

In the preoperative evaluation the anesthesiologist must define if the Fontan patient has a normal functioning or a failing Fontan, since it has important implications in the anesthetic management and in the perioperative care.

Medical history should focus on changes in health status, exercise capacity, hospital admissions, current medication and allergies. In addition to clinical examination, medical records, electrocardiography, chest X-ray, echocardiography, most recent catheterization, CMR imaging and laboratory data are invaluable to elucidate cardiac anatomy and the Fontan circuit, oxygen saturation, transpulmonary gradient and to assess ventricular function and valve regurgitation.

The physical exam of a well-functioning Fontan despite the univentricular pathology should be relatively unremarkable. The patient should be acyanotic, warm and well perfused. Precordial auscultation should be devoid of murmurs and peripheral arterial pulses are palpable. The arterial oxygen saturation is typically between 90% and 95% [5].

Failing Fontan physiology involves multiple organ systems: ventricular failure, hepatic disfunction, long lasting pleural effusions, pulmonary hypertension, PLE, plastic bronchitis. Symptoms indicative of a failing Fontan include dyspnea, fatigue, decline in exercise tolerance, weight gain or volume retention, palpitations, syncopal or pre-syncopal episodes, a new or worsening murmur, hepatomegaly, oxygen saturation below 90% and dyspnea [5]. Cardiomegaly and/or pleural effusions may herald a failing Fontan.

3.2.1 Cardiovascular evaluation

3.2.1.1 Functional status and exercise capacity

At peak exercise, a normal subject with a biventricular circuit can increase his CO by a factor of 5. In a patient with Fontan physiology, there is not physiologic mechanisms to allow for a similar increase in CO because the maximal mean venous pressure rarely reaches 30 mmHg, there is inability to power blood through the pulmonary vasculature and subsequent blood acceleration, and the reactivity of PVR is

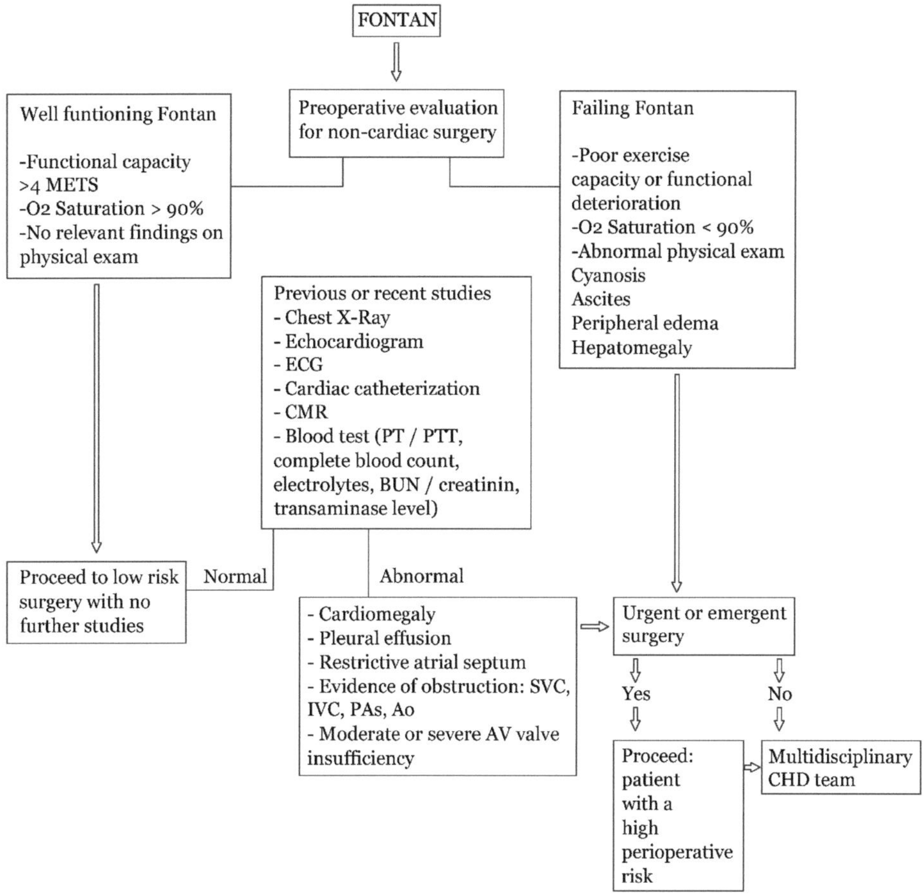

Figure 7.
Multisystem approach for Fontan patient preoperative evaluation.

attenuated or absent. These limitations combined, result in the diminished ability to augment CO in response to an increase in metabolic demand, therefore limiting the Fontan patient to perform exercise (**Figure 8**).

Under resting conditions, the CO of a Fontan patient is 70–80% of what it would normally be for age and body surface area. During physical activity the limitations of the Fontan circuit are substantially magnified; a small difference of CO at rest can become a much larger difference during activity. At the best Fontan, the output is mildly decreased at rest with moderate capacity to increase flow during moderate exercise. In the failing Fontan patient, the output is severely reduced at rest and barely augments during minimal exercise [2] (**Figure 9**).

Fontan patients have lived with less than ideal CO their entire lives and might not recognize symptoms or demonstrate overt manifestations of progressive decline in functional status until deterioration is quite advanced [6].

The New York Heart Association (NYHA) classification, originally established for patients with CHF, is now widely used in CHD. It represents a simple classification of exercise intolerance based on subjective symptoms. NYHA class does stratify patients, distinguishing patients with mild impairment from those with moderate or severe impairment of objective exercise capacity and the presence and severity of symptoms signify a worse objective exercise capacity. In the study of Diller et al., ACHD patients had exercise capacities as poor as those of patients with acquired

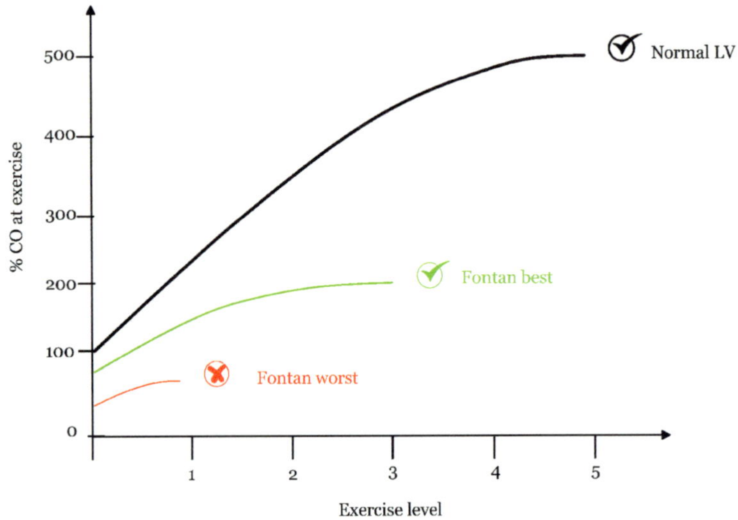

Figure 8.
CO and exercise level. At peak exercise, a normal subject with a biventricular circuit can increase his CO by a factor of 5. The Fontan patient has a diminished ability to augment CO in response to increased metabolic demand, and therefore limit the ability of a patient with a Fontan to perform exercise (CO, cardiac output; LV, left ventricle).

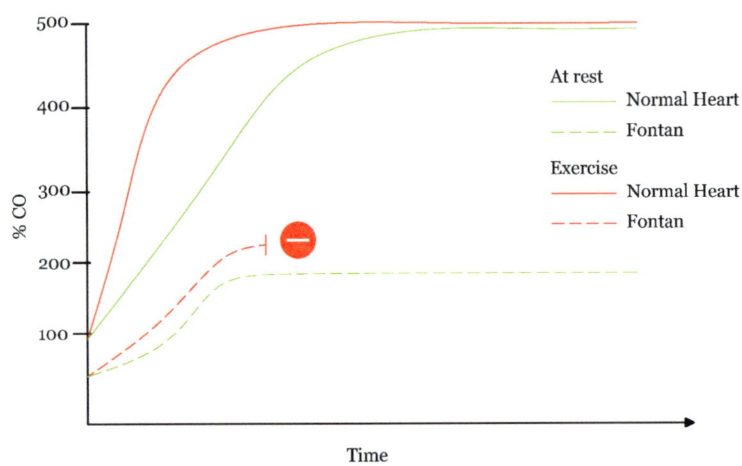

Figure 9.
Cardiac output in normal heart and the Fontan patient, during exercise and at rest. (CO, cardiac output).

CHF, even though the latter were much older [15]. Although NYHA class is used widely, the underlying criteria are subjective and the reproducibility is low.

In contrast to NYHA, cardiopulmonary exercise testing is the best way to assess exercise performance in ACHD patients, because it gives accurate, reproducible and quantifiable data on cardiac and respiratory performance, also allowing the assessment of unexpected deterioration. Most Fontan patients have undergone two or three re-operations, and this can lead to the development of restrictive lung defects in many patients. This finding, in addition to the restrictions in augmentation of the CO on exercise, contribute to a reduction in the measured peak oxygen uptake (peak VO_2), with average Fontan patients achieving a peak VO_2 of 60–70% that of age/sex/size-matched controls [7]. Longitudinal studies of late adolescents and young adults demonstrate this point well; as patients progress to late adolescence and early adulthood, exercise capacity tends to continue to decline by about 2.6% predicted per year [9, 16]. In many forms of CHD the cutoff for the development of symptoms of heart failure is an exercise capacity of 45–50% of the predicted value. Assuming a starting point of 65% predicted for age and at the onset of puberty in a Fontan patients, and calculating a decline of 2.6% per year thereafter, the cutoff of 45% predicted can be expected to be reached at the end of the second decade of life [2] and as typically occurs in the third decade of life, hospitalization rates and symptoms increase significantly [6, 16, 17]. Cardiopulmonary exercise testing can objectively quantify exercise tolerance and help guided therapy, therefore, peak VO_2 is an essential component of a tailored exercise and activity program [6].

In the Mayo Clinic cohort [10], 80% of the patients after the Fontan operation rated their current health as excellent, and a similar percentage of patients thought that their physical status was improved. This is consistent with previously reported data suggesting that patients tend to perceive themselves as having a higher functional status compared with control populations.

In the preoperative evaluation, it is important to recognize that NYHA class underestimates the true degree of exercise limitation in Fontan patients. It is likely that Fontan patients have made lifelong adaptations to their cardiovascular disease and its slow progression, so they are not aware of the true extent of their exercise intolerance and could consider themselves asymptomatic. The presence and severity of symptoms signify a worse objective exercise capacity in these patients [15].

3.2.1.2 Arrhythmias

Some factors contributing to arrhythmogenicity include systolic and diastolic dysfunction, atrioventricular valvular regurgitation, atrial enlargement, multiple cardiac procedures, myocardial fibrosis, APCs, intra-atrial tunnels and an abnormal array of atrial fibers. The incidence of late atrial tachyarrhythmias approaches 50% in the adult population after Fontan palliation and often results in decreased exercise capacity, fatigue and congestive heart failure [5–7, 10].

In the Mayo Clinic cohort [10], the diagnosis of new clinical arrhythmias during long term follow-up was present in 44% of the patients. Freedom of arrhythmia at 10, 20 and 30 years after the Fontan operation was 71%, 42% and 24% respectively. The majority of this patients had atrial fibrillation or flutter, and a smaller proportion presented, atrial tachycardia, re-entrant supra ventricular tachycardia and ventricular tachycardia.

Sinus node dysfunction is common in all Fontan variants, with prevalence rates as high as 40%. Sinoatrial dysfunction and bradyarrhythmias may necessitate placement of a dual-chamber pacemaker or resynchronization therapy [5].

In general, many strategies have been employed to reduce the arrhythmia burden, including oral antiarrhythmics and catheter ablation. A catheter-based ablation strategy has a considerably lower success rate in Fontan patients compared with other forms of CHD, with recurrences or new arrhythmias in approximately 50% within 4–5 years [6].

In the preoperative evaluation one should recognize the history of such arrhythmias and history electrophysiological procedures.

3.2.2 Pulmonary evaluation

In the preoperative evaluation determine the patient's saturation on room air, which in a well-functioning Fontan should be between 90% and 95%. In the case of desaturation, it is important elucidate the cause of hypoxemia (**Table 3**).

Low pulmonary venous saturation:
• Pleural effusions
• Pulmonary arteriovenous malformations
• Intrinsic lung disease
• Plastic bronchitis
Right-to-left shunt:
• Veno-venous collateral vessels
• Persistent fenestration
• Baffle leak

Table 3.
Common sources of hypoxemia in the Fontan patient.

Persistent or recurrent pleural effusions can be a source of hypoxemia in Fontan patients. Systemic oxygen desaturation can also be found because of intrapulmonary shunting due to arteriovenous malformations. The unequal distribution of hepatic blood flow to the pulmonary system is the most accepted etiology. Less hepatic blood flow to the pulmonary vasculature makes it more prone to developing arteriovenous malformations [5].

As pointed before, most Fontan patients have undergone at least two or three open chest procedures and may have undergone a thoracotomy that leads to a restrictive lung defect. Nearly half of all ACHD patients have lung disease with a primarily restrictive pattern, which represents an independent predictor for mortality [18]. The etiology is multifactorial: intrinsic causes of restrictive lung disease range from decrease in the pulmonary blood flow, development of arteriovenous malformations at the level of the lung and the long standing persistent abnormal physiology that contributes to the changes in the pulmonary vascular bed. Extrinsic causes are related to the multiple re-operations, congenital chest wall and spinal deformities, preexisting muscle weakness, all having an effect in the pulmonary mechanics. Other contributing factors as extended mechanical ventilation due to critical illness during childhood, chronic aspiration, acquire muscle weakness, and poor nutrition, can result in impaired pulmonary function [18].

Plastic bronchitis is a rare complication reported in less than 1–2% of Fontan patients. It is characterized by bronchial casts, with potential for airway obstruction. Segmental airway obstruction can result in regional atelectasis and hypoxemia. Dyspnea, chronic cough, and recurrent expectoration of rubber airway casts are characteristic of this disorder. Plastic bronchitis can be life-threatening on presentation [6].

Another source of hypoxemia in Fontan patients include persistent right-to-left shunting. Maintaining adequate preload for the SV is challenging in the Fontan patient, and it relies on a number of "auto-regulatory" phenomena, including the development of veno-venous collateral vessels that pass from the systemic veins to the pulmonary venous circulation shunting deoxygenated blood directly into the oxygenated pulmonary venous system or the common atrium. The downside to maintaining an adequate preload and CO is the profound cyanosis that can be worsened by physical exertion (**Figure 6**).

The strategy employed in many centers is a catheter based embolization of these vessels. The impact on the symptoms or survival has not been determined, and further reduction in oxygen saturation post-procedure, suggest a high recurrence rate [5, 7].

Systemic-to-PA collaterals are a frequent finding in cyanotic Fontan patients. Left alone, these collateral vessels may result in pulmonary hypertension and failure of the Fontan circulation.

3.2.3 Hematologic evaluation

Hypercoagulability and hypocoagulability both are more prevalent in patients with Fontan physiology [18].

After the Fontan operation, patients have been reported to have numerous clotting abnormalities including deficiencies of protein C, protein S and antithrombin III. Hypercoagulability combined with decreased CO, a nonpulsatile low flow state to the pulmonary circulation, a high incidence of atrial arrhythmias and the presence of prosthetic material, contribute to a higher risk for thrombus formation in the Fontan patient [9].

Some studies have reported a rate of thrombus formation of up to 20% in patients after a Fontan procedure and they are a source of significant morbidity and mortality [5, 9]. The incidence of thromboemboli after the extracardiac cavopulmonary connection is estimated to be 7.1% at 10 years after Fontan completion. This can result in pulmonary emboli, systemic emboli through a patent fenestration and systemic thrombi in the atria, PA stump or rudimentary ventricle [9].

Approximately 10% of patients within the first 5 years after Fontan palliation, develop thrombotic occlusion of central veins, this can result in pulmonary emboli and in SVC obstruction. Clinicians should not assume patency or availability of venous access for central monitoring of the subclavian, internal jugular or femoral vessels. The anesthesiologist relies on cardiac catheterization reports and Doppler ultrasound to assess vascular patency of the venous and arterial tree [5]. Many patients are on anticoagulants or aspirin, especially those with thrombosis history or with a failing Fontan with any of the following manifestations: ventricular failure, hepatic disfunction, long lasting pleural effusions, pulmonary hypertension, PLE, and plastic bronchitis.

3.2.4 Neurologic evaluation

The reported incidence of stroke ranges from 3% to 20%. Cerebral vascular accidents have been reported in adult patients with Fontan physiology secondary to atrial arrhythmias, hematologic derangements and systemic embolic events [5].

3.2.5 Hepatic and gastrointestinal evaluation

Fontan physiology, in particular, with the multitude of insults from persistent congestive hepatopathy, hypoxia, and ischemic hepatitis, has a high incidence of liver dysfunction [18].

There is growing recognition of the deleterious effects of systemic venous hypertension on hepatic function and the development of fibrosis, cirrhosis and hepatocellular carcinoma.

PLE is a cardinal sign of failing Fontan palliation. Pleural effusions with associated decreases in oxygen saturation, peripheral edema, ascites, malabsorption and loss of immunoglobulins are consistent findings in patients with PLE. Hypoalbuminemia, decreased total protein and stool positive for alpha 1-antitrypsin confirm the diagnosis [5, 7].

In the Mayo Clinic cohort [10] was found that although the Fontan procedure has improved overall survival in patients with SV, various events impact long-term survival, including diagnosis of PLE. The overall incidence of PLE in this study was 9%. Overall mortality in the PLE cohort was 72% during 7 + – 7.4 years of follow-up. Survival at 5, 10, and 20 years after PLE diagnosis was 50%, 35% and 19%, respectively [10].

3.2.6 Renal evaluation

ACHD patients have a prevalence of renal dysfunction 18 to 35 fold higher compared to the general population. Renal dysfunction is seen in 50% of Fontan patients, including a 15% presenting with severe reduction of glomerular filtration rate [19].

3.2.7 Imaging

Preoperatively the use of recent or previous imaging studies allows the proper assessment of the Fontan cardiac function, pathway and vascular anatomy.

Chest radiography can present with abnormalities consistent with a failing Fontan, including cardiomegaly, pleural effusion and pulmonary edema.

To evaluate systolic and diastolic ventricular function is important to perform a preoperative TTE or TEE, it also evaluates atrioventricular valve function, the presence of an open fenestration and detects intracardiac thrombi.

Cardiac catheterization evaluates the Fontan hemodynamics measuring CAP, CVP, ventricular end-diastolic pressure, sampling blood along the vessels and chambers to determine their saturations and, CI calculation with the Fick Method. A high preoperative CAP suggests poor ventricular function, atrioventricular valve dysfunction or the presence of aortopulmonary collaterals. Isolated high CVP with low CAP reflects increased PVR or an obstruction along the Fontan pathway.

Cardiac catheterization can also allow the measurement of pressure gradients of obstructive lesions in the vena cava, pulmonary vessels and across the atrial septal defect. It is also used to assess the presence of right-to-left shunts causing desaturation as baffle leaks, fenestrations, decompressing veno-venous collateral vessels, pulmonary arteriovenous malformations and systemic to pulmonary collaterals. Catheter-based interventions may be required to alleviate obstruction in the Fontan pathway, for managing profound cyanosis or for stenting of branch PA stenosis or venous pathway obstruction [7].

CMR imaging is increasingly used in assessing anatomy, flow, and function in the Fontan patient without a pacemaker [5, 7]. It is used to asses Fontan pathway flow, it also assess pulmonary venous return to exclude obstruction. In addition it can provide with an accurate assessment of the ventricular function and assessment of the branch PAs, and in the ventricular outflow pathway it can exclude recoarctation or narrowing [7].

Urgent and emergent noncardiac surgeries or invasive procedures should not be delayed for sophisticated imaging in the preoperative evaluation, but the anesthesiologist should be aware of the previous studies and the actual anatomy of the patient.

4. Intraoperative management

Although there are guidelines for the perioperative management of patients with CHD undergoing noncardiac surgery [14, 18, 20–22], these recommendations are based on experience and expert opinion. The diversity of structural malformations in CHD, each with specific physiologic perturbations, hemodynamic consequences, and functional limitations, makes the development of general guidelines for perioperative management challenging [13].

4.1 Hemodynamic monitoring

Standard American Society of Anesthesiologists (ASA) intraoperative monitoring is often adequate for patients with a well-functioning Fontan, particularly for procedures in which minimal hemodynamic derangements or fluid shifts are expected.

For the failing Fontan patient or well-functioning Fontan patient presenting for more complex surgical procedures, intra-arterial blood pressure monitoring is useful for beat-to-beat monitoring of blood pressure and blood sampling to asses sufficient systemic perfusion and adequate balance in oxygen delivery and consumption by measuring laboratory values such as lactate levels and central venous oxygenation [5, 18].

Upper-extremity blood pressure (noninvasive and radial arterial catheters) should be measured in the arm opposite to a previous Blalock-Taussig shunt (subclavian artery-to-PA) to avoid falsely low blood pressure measurements [5].

It should be noted that CVP actually reflects mean PA pressure (MPAP) in Fontan patients.

Intraoperative placement of transcutaneous defibrillator pads is prudent in patients with a history of arrhythmias [5].

4.2 Vascular access

Regarding vascular access, abnormal vascular anatomy of the initial CHD, post-surgical changes, multiple vascular interventions, and prior thrombus formation can pose significant challenges when patients are in need of vascular access [5].

Even though upper central venous access is possible in patients with Fontan circulation, exact knowledge of vascular anatomy is crucial for venous cannulation. Venous mapping can be highly valuable before any intervention, and access obtained by interventional radiologists under direct fluoroscopic guidance may be required. A graph depicting which vascular access is patent in a particular patient should be readily available to the care team in order to avoid difficulty in placing lines in an emergency [18].

Another consideration when obtaining and maintaining vascular access is the risk of paradoxic emboli in the presence of right-to-left or bidirectional shunting through the post-surgical fenestration. Entrained air and dislodged thrombotic or infectious material can lead to paradoxic emboli and to infarction of brain, gut, kidney, and other end organs [18]. Before the administration of intravenous fluids or medications, all air must be evacuated meticulously and filtered to avoid systemic air embolism and use of air filters can mitigate the risk of accidental air entrainment [5, 18].

It is recommended that central venous catheters be removed as soon as possible to avoid thrombotic complications [5].

4.3 Anesthetic goals

There are important anesthetic considerations for the patient with Fontan physiology.

4.3.1 Maintenance an optimal transpulmonary gradient

The mainstay of anesthetic management is to maintain an optimal transpulmonary gradient in order to achieve an adequate pulmonary blood flow and CO. The Fontan (CVP = MPAP) is typically 10 to 15 mmHg with a transpulmonary gradient of 7 mmHg. It is helpful to determine CAP values from the preoperative catheterization because the anesthesiologist will not monitor this value in the operating room.

4.3.2 Differential diagnosis of desaturation

The differential diagnosis of acute oxygen desaturation in the intraoperative period may include factors unique to the Fontan patient.

Right-to-left shunts become important causes of hypoxemia. Acute elevation of PVR may cause right-to-left shunting across a fenestration or a baffle leak with the consequent drop in the saturation of the patient. PVR may be decreased acutely with hyperventilation (pCO_2 30 mmHg or pH 7.45) and increasing concentrations of oxygen. Usual sources of hypoxemia in the perioperative period such as endobronchial intubation, bronchospasm, and atelectasis always should be considered.

4.3.3 Respiratory management

The circulatory arrangement of the Fontan amplifies the effects of respiratory mechanics upon venous return. Negative intra-thoracic pressure augments the antegrade flow from the SVC, IVC, and hepatic venous circulation into the pulmonary arterial tree. The work of breathing is a significant additional energy source to the circulation in these patients. Normal negative pressure inspiration has been shown to increase pulmonary blood flow in patients after the TCPC [3]. Physiologically there is a correlation between total hepatic venous flow and respiration. During inspiration there is marked increase in hepatic venous contribution to the total venous return, due to a dual effect on venous pressure and compression of the liver by diaphragmatic decent. The liver acts as a sump of blood which can be drawn upon during inspiration [3].

Magnetic resonance flow measurements have shown that approximately 30% of the CO can be directly attributed to the work of breathing in patients after the TCPC [3]. In Fontan patients, inspiration resulted in increased ventricular filling at rest and during exercise [23].

The opposite happens with positive pressure ventilation (PPV). It has long been known that increasing levels of positive end-expiratory pressure (PEEP) during PPV are adverse to the Fontan circulation. The available data suggests a linear relationship between mean airway pressure and CI in these patients: the higher the mean airway pressure, the lower CI [3]. This can be explained by the effect of lung volumes on PVR, since both over-distention and collapse of alveoli, result in increases in PVR.

The management of these patients should therefore be directed towards minimizing mean airway pressure when these patients are being ventilated for cardiac and noncardiac procedures. Also, an early postoperative restoration of normal negative pressure ventilation can be beneficial in these patients.

Adjustments to minimize positive intra-thoracic pressure can be made using minimal PEEP, smaller tidal volumes, pressure-regulated ventilatory modes, or spontaneous ventilation with minimal pressure support [18], and avoid prolonged Valsalva maneuvers. One should maintain these patients with the minimum mean airway pressure compatible with normal oxygenation and adequate alveolar ventilation.

A sound strategy when using PPV would be to adjust ventilatory parameters that allows to achieve the lowest mean airway pressure, moderate alkalosis (pH 7.45, pCO_2 35 mmHg), and one that reduces the risk of atelectasis. Fontan patients have tolerated PPV with minimal hemodynamic effects as long as proper ventilatory settings are used. Furthermore, it has been proposed that monitored anesthesia care without adequate ventilation may be more detrimental than the physiologic effects of PPV per se [5].

4.3.4 Circulatory management

Fontan patients pose a particular clinical challenge for the anesthesiologist due to their abnormal physiology and high risk for adverse events. Pre-existing chronic end-organ dysfunction makes these patients susceptible to acute exacerbation or organ failure [18]. Information of baseline cardiac function and hemodynamics from prior heart catheterizations can provide reference filling pressures to minimize the risk of over-resuscitation or under-resuscitation.

Fontan physiology patients are very sensitive to changes in preload, and high PPV settings can exacerbate hemodynamic instability as was explained before. Acute hypovolemia or vasodilation during critical illness can result in significant hypotension.

The effect of vasoconstrictors in augmenting preload in Fontan physiology is unclear because the compliance of the venous capacity system is reduced, and also an increase in ventricular afterload, due to arterial vasoconstriction, can decrease forward flow [18]. Hypervolemia due to excessive fluid resuscitation or chronically in the failing Fontan, can result in a reduced CO due to a decreased pressure gradient between systemic arterial and venous capacity system. Global congestion can lead to impaired pulmonary blood flow and right-sided congestion with subsequent pulmonary edema, kidney and hepatic dysfunction.

Finding the optimal volume status that balances adequate preload, venous congestion and organ perfusion could be challenging and requires vigilance and significant experience with these complex pathophysiologic states. Defining the end point of fluid administration (Blood components, Crystalloids) should be a balance of the risks and benefits of resuscitation. It is important to have the baseline pressures, hemoglobin level, signs of inadequate oxygen delivery, and concurrent factors affecting hemodynamics in order to decide how much and which fluid requires a particular patient [18].

Universally important applicable components when managing hemodynamics in these patients include maintaining adequate heart rate and intrinsic sympathetic tone, avoiding increases in PVR, and limiting harm from elevated intra-thoracic or intra-abdominal pressures [18].

Risks associated with medical intervention especially adrenergic agents are exacerbation of arrhythmias.

Low-cardiac-output syndrome will manifest as hypotension, elevated CVP, metabolic and lactic acidosis, and low urine output in the intraoperative period. Pharmacologically improving ventricular compliance lowers the CAP and increases the transpulmonary gradient without raising CVP. Milrinone, with its lusitropic and pulmonary vasodilatory properties, is well suited for the Fontan patient. Because systolic performance is not generally the primary issue in the Fontan circulation, the role of inotropic agents is often limited, and lowering the SVR while maintaining preload can be challenging. Inodilators increase the contractility of the SV, but may not result in clinically significant more CO. There may be a role for inotropes in the Fontan patient with significant ventricular dysfunction but in general the role of these agents is limited [2].

5. Conclusions

- Since prognosis of patients with univentricular heart has improved significantly in recent decades, this has resulted in the general anesthesiologist being able to meet at some point in his professional practice with this type of patients, whether to perform a noncardiovascular diagnostic or therapeutic procedure or noncardiac surgery. Therefore, the anesthesiologist must have an appropriate knowledge of Fontan's anatomy and physiology as well as those patients with failed Fontan in order to provide them with a correct preoperative evaluation and an adequate intraoperative and postoperative management, and to obtain the best results, thus achieving a better survival and quality of life in this population group.

- The differentiation between a patient with Fontan palliation in a compensated state versus the failing Fontan patient is one of the goals of the preoperative evaluation since the latter has a higher perioperative risk.

- Fontan patients may present with a multisystemic compromise and this poses challenges in the intraoperative management of noncardiac surgical or invasive procedures.

- Causes of intraoperative hypoxemia may be different from a patient with biventricular physiology. Situations unique for the Fontan patient include right-to-left shunting through the fenestration and the presence of veno-venous collateral vessels.

- There is evidence that circulatory failure rather than ventricular failure is most important in the Fontan patient. In the failing Fontan one should rule out any problem in the Fontan circuit.

- Finally, this chapter covers a series of information with the purpose of facilitating a timely and complete orientation of univentricular patients in the stage of Fontan palliation, since these imply a challenge in professional practice.

Conflict of interest

No conflicts of interest to declare.

Thanks/other declarations

Especial thanks to Ignacio Granados Vega for his wonderful illustrations.

Author details

Yamile Muñoz[1*], María José Sáenz[2] and Renzo Cifuentes[3]

1 Department of Anesthesia, Clínica Cardio VID, Medellín, Colombia

2 Department of Anesthesia, National Children Hospital, San José, Costa Rica

3 Department of Surgery, Division of Thoracic Transplantation and MCS, Miller School of Medicine, University of Miami, USA

*Address all correspondence to: yamilemp@yahoo.com

References

[1] Faraoni D, Zurakowski D, Vo D, Goobie SM, Yuki K, Brown ML, et al. Post-operative outcomes in children with and without congenital heart disease undergoing noncardiac surgery. Journal of American College of Cardiology. 2016;**67**(7):793-801. DOI: 10.1016/j.jacc.2015.11.057

[2] Gewillig M, Goldberg DJ. Failure of the fontan circulation. Heart Failure Clinics. 2014;**10**(1):105-116

[3] Redington A. The physiology of the Fontan circulation. Progress in Pediatric Cardiology. 2006;**22**(2):179-186. ISSN: 1058-9813. DOI: 10.1016/j.ppedcard.2006.07.007. (http://www.sciencedirect.com/science/article/pii/S1058981306000518)

[4] Davies RR, Pizarro C. Decision-making for surgery in the Management of Patients with Univentricular heart. Frontiers in Pediatrics. 2015;**3**:61. DOI: 10.3389/fped.2015.00061. eCollection 2015. Review

[5] Eagle SS, Daves SM. The adult with Fontan physiology: Systematic approach to perioperative management for noncardiac surgery. Journal of Cardiothoracic and Vascular Anesthesia. 2011 Apr;**25**(2):320-334. DOI: 10.1053/j.jvca.2010.12.003. Review

[6] Mondésert B, Marcotte F, Mongeon FP, Dore A, Mercier LA, Ibrahim R, et al. Fontan circulation: Success or failure? The Canadian Journal of Cardiology. 2013 Jul;**29**(7):811-820. DOI: 10.1016/j.cjca.2012.12.009

[7] Clift P, Celermajer D. Managing adult Fontan patients: Where do we stand? European Respiratory Review. 2016 Dec;**25**(142):438-450. DOI: 10.1183/16000617.0091-2016

[8] Vaughn G, Moore J, Lamberti J, Canter C. Management of the failing Fontan: Medical, interventional and surgical treatment. Progress in Pediatric Cardiology. 2016;**43**:51-56. ISSN: 1058-9813. (http://www.sciencedirect.com/science/article/pii/S1058981316300510). DOI: 10.1016/j.ppedcard.2016.07.007

[9] John AS. Fontan repair of single ventricle physiology: Consequences of a unique physiology and possible treatment options. Cardiology Clinics. 2015;**33**(4):559-569, viii. DOI: 10.1016/j.ccl.2015.07.010

[10] Pundi KN, Johnson JN, Dearani JA, Pundi KN, Li Z, Hinck CA, et al. 40-year follow-up after the Fontan operation: Long-term outcomes of 1,052 patients. Journal of the American College of Cardiology. 2015;**66**(15):1700-1710. DOI: 10.1016/j.jacc.2015.07.065

[11] Griffiths ER, Kaza AK, Wyler von Ballmoos MC, Loyola H, Valente AM, Blume ED, et al. Evaluating failing Fontans for heart transplantation: Predictors of death. Annals of Thoracic Surgery. 2009;**88**(2):558-563; discussion 563-4. DOI: 10.1016/j.athoracsur.2009.03.085

[12] Hebson CL, McCabe NM, Elder RW, Mahle WT, McConnell M, Kogon BE, et al. Hemodynamic phenotype of the failing Fontan in an adult population. The American Journal of Cardiology. 2013;**112**(12):1943-1947. DOI: 10.1016/j.amjcard.2013.08.023

[13] Faraoni D, Vo D, Nasr VG, DiNardo JA. Development and validation of a risk stratification score for children with congenital heart disease undergoing noncardiac surgery. Anesthesia and Analgesia. 2016;**123**(4):824-830. DOI: 10.1213/ANE.0000000000001500

[14] Stout KK, Daniels CJ, Aboulhosn JA, Bozkurt B, Broberg CS, Colman JM,

et al. 2018 AHA/ACC guideline for the Management of Adults with Congenital Heart Disease: A report of the American College of Cardiology/American Heart Association task force on clinical practice guidelines. Circulation. 2019;**139**(14):e698-e800. DOI: 10.1161/CIR.0000000000000603

[15] Diller GP, Dimopoulos K, Okonko D, Li W, Babu-Narayan SV, Broberg CS, et al. Exercise intolerance in adult congenital heart disease: Comparative severity, correlates, and prognostic implication. Circulation. 2005;**112**(6):828-835. DOI: 10.1161/CIRCULATIONAHA.104.529800

[16] Valente AM, Lewis M, Vaziri SM, Bautista-Hernandez V, Harmon A, Kim Y, et al. Outcomes of adolescents and adults undergoing primary Fontan procedure. The American Journal of Cardiology. 2013;**112**(12):1938-1942. DOI: 10.1016/j.amjcard.2013.08.021

[17] Khairy P, Fernandes SM, Mayer JE Jr, Triedman JK, Walsh EP, Lock JE, et al. Long-term survival, modes of death, and predictors of mortality in patients with Fontan surgery. Circulation. 2008;**117**(1):85-92. DOI: 10.1161/CIRCULATIONAHA.107.738559

[18] Kratzert WB, Boyd EK, Schwarzenberger JC. Management of the Critically ill Adult with Congenital Heart Disease. Journal of Cardiothoracic and Vascular Anesthesia. 2018;**32**(4):1682-1700. DOI: 10.1053/j.jvca. 2017.11.025

[19] Dimopoulos K, Diller GP, Koltsida E, Pijuan-Domenech A, Papadopoulou SA, Babu-Narayan SV, et al. Prevalence, predictors, and prognostic value of renal dysfunction in adults with congenital heart disease. Circulation. 2008;**117**(18):2320-2328. DOI: 10.1161/CIRCULATIONAHA.107.734921

[20] Smith S, Walker A. Anaesthetic implications of congenital heart disease for children undergoing non-cardiac surgery. Anaesthesia & Intensive Care Medicine. 2018;**19**(8):414-420. ISSN: 1472-0299. (http://www.sciencedirect.com/science/article/pii/S1472029918301103). DOI: 10.1016/j.mpaic.2018.04.011

[21] Cannesson M, Earing MG, Collange V, Kersten JR. Anesthesia for noncardiac surgery in adults with congenital heart disease. Anesthesiology. 2009 Aug;**111**(2):432-440. DOI: 10.1097/ALN.0b013e3181ae51a6

[22] Baehner T, Ellerkmann RK. Anesthesia in adults with congenital heart disease. Current Opinion in Anaesthesiology. 2017 Jun;**30**(3):418-425. DOI: 10.1097/ACO.0000000000000468 Review

[23] Van De Bruaene A, Claessen G, La Gerche A, Kung E, Marsden A, De Meester P, et al. Effect of respiration on cardiac filling at rest and during exercise in Fontan patients: A clinical and computational modeling study. International Journal of Cardiology/Heart & Vasculature. 2015;**9**:100-108. DOI: 10.1016/j.ijcha.2015.08.002 eCollection 2015 Dec 7

Chapter 7

Fontan Operation: A Comprehensive Review

P. Syamasundar Rao

Abstract

Since the first description of the Fontan operation in the early 1970s, a number of modifications have been introduced and currently staged, total cavopulmonary connection with fenestration has become the most commonly used multistage surgery in diverting the vena caval blood flow into the lungs. The existing ventricle, whether it is left or right, is utilized to supply systemic circuit. During Stage I, palliative surgery is performed, usually at presentation in the neonatal period/early infancy, on the basis of pathophysiology of the cardiac defect. During Stage II, a bidirectional Glenn procedure is undertaken in which the superior vena caval flow is diverted into the lungs at an approximate age of 6 months. During Stage IIIA, the blood flow from the inferior vena cava (IVC) is rerouted into the pulmonary arteries, typically by an extra-cardiac conduit along with a fenestration, generally around 2 years of age. During Stage IIIB, the fenestration is closed by transcatheter methodology 6–12 months after Stage IIIA. The evolution of Fontan concepts, the indications for Fontan surgery, and the results of old and current types of Fontan operation form the focus of this review.

Keywords: Fontan operation, bidirectional Glenn procedure, modified Blalock-Taussig shunt, pulmonary artery banding, Norwood procedure, Sano shunt, extra-cardiac conduit, fenestrated Fontan, tricuspid atresia, double-inlet left ventricle, hypoplastic left heart syndrome, unbalanced atrioventricular septal defect

1. Introduction

Following the initial description of the physiologically corrective operation for tricuspid atresia by Fontan and Baudet [1] and Kreutzer and his associates [2] almost simultaneously, such surgery was widely adapted by most pediatric cardiologists and pediatric cardiac surgeons. This concept of bypassing the right ventricle (RV) was further extended to manage other cardiac defects with a functionally single ventricle.

The original surgery as described by Fontan and Baudet [1] consisted of (1) end-to-end anastomosis of superior vena cava (SVC) with the right pulmonary artery (PA) (classical Glenn procedure [3]), (2) connection of the separated right PA to the right atrium (RA) either directly or through an aortic homograft, (3) closure of the defect in the atrial septum, (4) insertion of a pulmonary valve homograft into the orifice of the inferior vena cava (IVC), and (5) ligation of the main PA, to entirely bypass the RV. On the basis of the procedures performed, one must infer that Fontan's concept was to use the right atrium as a pumping chamber;

IntechOpen

therefore, he inserted a prosthetic valve into the IVC and right atrial-pulmonary artery junction.

On the contrary, Kreutzer et al. [2] anastomosed the right atrial appendage to the PA directly or by a pulmonary homograft and closed the ASD. Neither a Glenn procedure was performed nor a prosthetic valve was inserted in the IVC. Kreutzer's view appears to be that the RA does not function as a pump and that the left ventricle functions as a suction pump in the system.

The surgical procedure as generally performed appears to shadow Kreutzer's principle, and consequently, I have used the term "Fontan-Kreutzer operation" to describe this procedure [4–8]. However, because of priority of publication and more common usage in the literature, I will use the term "Fontan operation" in this chapter.

In this review, I will discuss the evolution of the Fontan concepts, the indications for Fontan operation, the Fontan procedure as used currently, and the results of old and current types of Fontan.

2. Evolution of the Fontan operation

A number of modifications of the aforementioned surgery were made by these [1, 2] and other groups of investigators [9, 10] in the field. In this section, these concepts/procedures will be reviewed.

2.1 Initial surgical modifications

During the first 20 years after Fontan's [1] and Kruetzer's [2] description of the procedure, a number of modifications of the surgery were undertaken by several surgeons, as extensively reviewed and referenced elsewhere [9, 10]. In general, there was a consensus that there is no need for a classic Glenn anastomosis and that a prosthetic valve is not necessary in the IVC. Detailed review of these papers revealed that four major types of Fontan operations were being performed for physiologic correction of tricuspid atresia. These include (1) RA-PA anastomosis, direct or through a non-valved conduit; (2) RA-PA anastomosis through a valved conduit; (3) RA-RV anastomosis, direct or non-valved anastomosis; and (4) RA-RV anastomosis through a valved conduit.

In order to understand the advantages of one operation over the other, 17 papers published as of December 1990 that have documented adequate information to evaluate mortality and reoperation rates for each of the four types of Fontan surgery were reviewed. Pooled data from these 17 articles and statistical comparisons were presented in Tables I–IV for the interested reader [9]. This analysis revealed that atriopulmonary (RA-PA) connection appears to be better than atrioventricular (RA-RV) anastomosis and direct connection is better than valved or non-valved conduit anastomosis. Nevertheless, atrioventricular valved (homograft) conduit anastomosis appears to have advantages of (1) restoring a four-valved, four-chambered, biventricular heart and (2) lower right atrial pressure than with atriopulmonary connection. Based on these data [9, 10], the following conclusions were drawn: (1) direct atriopulmonary connection for children with tricuspid atresia with normally related great arteries and a small (<30% of normal) right ventricle without trabecular right ventricular component and for patients who had tricuspid atresia with transposition of the great arteries and (2) atrioventricular valved (homograft) conduit anastomosis for patients with tricuspid atresia and normally related great arteries but with a right ventricular size greater than 30% of normal and a trabecular right ventricular component [9, 10].

2.2 Other developments

2.2.1 Bidirectional Glenn procedure (cavopulmonary anastomosis)

Bidirectional cavopulmonary anastomosis is a modified version of classic Glenn procedure in which the upper end of the divided SVC is anastomosed end to side to the right PA without disconnecting the latter from the main PA. Thus, the SVC blood is diverted into both the right and left PAs, justifying the term, "bidirectional."

Experimental bidirectional cavopulmonary anastomosis was first studied by Haller et al. [11] in animal models, and its first clinical use was described by Azzolina et al. [12] in 1972. Other investigators [13–17] later applied this technique to palliate complex heart defects with decreased pulmonary blood flow. Hemodynamic advantages of the bidirectional Glenn procedure are improvement of effective pulmonary blood flow, decrease in total pulmonary blood flow, and reduction of left ventricular volume overloading. In addition, preservation of continuity of the pulmonary artery is an added advantage and may help facilitate a low-risk Fontan procedure. When both right and left SVCs are present, bilateral bidirectional Glenn shunts should be performed, especially if the bridging innominate vein is absent or small. Based on our own experience and that published in the literature [13–17], the author recommended serious consideration in employing bidirectional cavopulmonary anastomosis as an interim palliative procedure for patients who are at an increased risk for the Fontan procedure [9, 10].

2.2.2 Lateral tunnel

Puga et al. [18] positioned a patch inside the right atrium to divert the IVC blood into the PAs; they had good results in the 12 patients that they used this technique. This was later called lateral tunnel and was widely used until extra-cardiac conduits came into vogue.

2.2.3 Total cavopulmonary connection

To better understand the valve-less atriopulmonary anastomosis type of Fontan, de Leval et al. [19] performed hydrodynamic studies and found that (1) the right atrium is not an efficient pump in non-valved atriopulmonary connections, (2) pulsations in a non-valved circulation truly generate turbulence with consequent decrease in net flow, and (3) energy losses occur in the non-pulsatile chambers, corners, and obstructions. In an attempt to address these deficiencies, they developed a procedure which they named "total cavopulmonary connection." In this procedure, they connected the divided SVC, end to side, to the undivided right pulmonary artery (bidirectional Glenn), and the IVC blood is diverted through a composite intra-atrial tunnel (with the use of posterior wall of the right atrium as posterior wall of the tunnel) into the cardiac end of the divided superior vena cava, which in turn was connected to the PA. They felt that technical simplicity, maintenance of low right atrial and coronary sinus pressure, and reduction of risk of atrial thrombus formation are advantages of this type of operation. They performed this procedure on 20 patients and observed two early deaths and one late death. Postoperative hemodynamic studies were performed in 10 of the survivors which indicated good results. They recommended this type of operation for patients with a non-hypertrophied right atrium. While the total cavopulmonary connection was initially devised for patients with complex atrial anatomy and/or systemic venous anomalies, it has since been used extensively for all types of cardiac anatomy with one functioning ventricle and irrespective of venous anomalies.

Subsequent experimental studies by Sharma and his associates [20] indicated that complete or minimal offset between the orifices of the SVC and IVC into the right pulmonary artery decreases energy losses.

2.2.4 Extra-cardiac conduit

Marcelletti et al. [21, 22] used an interposition extra-cardiac conduit from the IVC to the PA in place of lateral tunnel used in total cavopulmonary connection in 1990. Subsequently, most surgeons adopted this modification of total cavopulmonary connection, and currently extra-cardiac conduits are used in most Fontan operations.

2.2.5 Staged Fontan

Since the vast majority of patients requiring Fontan operation present as neonates or in the early infancy, palliative procedures are performed at the time of presentation, and subsequently (at 12–18 months of age) the Fontan operation is undertaken. A considerable mortality (~16%) was seen with primary Fontan surgery, largely related to the impact of rapid changes in ventricular geometry and development of ventricular diastolic dysfunction. The concept of further staging the procedure by performing bidirectional Glenn procedure around 6 months of age followed by final Fontan between 12 and 18 months of age was introduced in early 1990s [23, 24]. Performing the Fontan procedure in stages appears to decrease overall mortality, most likely related to improving the ventricular function by correction of the afterload mismatch that is associated with one-stage Fontan procedure. At the current time, most centers prefer staged Fontan with bidirectional Glenn initially, followed later by extra-cardiac conduit diversion of the inferior vena caval blood into the PA.

2.2.6 Fenestrated Fontan operation

In 1978, Choussat et al. proposed several criteria for performing Fontan operation [25]. Many cardiologists and surgeons have modified these criteria. Patients not meeting these criteria were deemed to be at a higher risk for a poor prognosis following a Fontan operation than patients who are within the limits of the set criteria. For the high-risk group, several investigators have proposed the concept of leaving a small atrial septal defect (ASD) open to facilitate decompression of the right atrium [26–28]. Laks et al. advocated closure of the atrial defect by constricting the preplaced suture in the postoperative period [28], while Bridges et al. [27] used a transcatheter closure method at a later date.

Higher cardiac output and significant decreases in the postoperative pleural effusions and systemic venous congestion were noted after a fenestrated Fontan procedure. In addition, the duration of hospitalization appears to have decreased. Nonetheless, these beneficial effects are at the expense of mild arterial hypoxemia and potential for paradoxical embolism.

While the fenestrated Fontan procedure was initially designed for patients at high risk for Fontan surgery, it has since been used in patients with modest or even low risk. Although rare, reports of cerebrovascular or other systemic arterial embolic events occurring after a fenestrated Fontan operation tend to contraindicate the use of fenestrations in patients with low or usual risk. In following years, fenestrated Fontan have been routinely used at most institutions. Some data indicate that routine fenestration is not necessary [29].

2.2.7 Device closure of Fontan fenestration

Patients who have undergone a fenestrated Fontan operation or patients who have a residual atrial defect, despite correction, may have clinically significant right-to-left shunt causing varying degrees of hypoxemia. These residual defects should be closed not only to address arterial desaturation but also for prevention of paradoxical embolism [30, 31]. Although two types of fenestration closure, namely, constriction of the preplaced suture in the postoperative period [26, 28] and device closure later [27] were described, device closure is opted at most institutions. Closure of such defects can be performed by using transcatheter techniques [32–35]. The procedure is usually performed 6–12 months following fenestrated Fontan procedure. Although a number of devices have been used in the past [32–35], at the present time, Amplatzer septal occluders are the most commonly used devices to accomplish such closures.

3. Indications for Fontan operation

The indications for opting for a Fontan operation are patients who have one functioning ventricle. At first, patients with tricuspid atresia were selected for this procedure [1, 2]. Shortly thereafter, patients with double-inlet left (single) ventricle were added to the indications for Fontan [36]. Following description of surgical palliation of hypoplastic left heart syndrome (HLHS) by Norwood et al. [37, 38] in the early 1980s, HLHS became the major lesion requiring Fontan operation. Subsequently, mitral atresia (with normal aortic root), unbalanced atrioventricular septal defects (AVSDs), pulmonary atresia with intact ventricular septum with markedly hypoplastic right ventricle, and other complex heart defects with one functioning ventricle were selected for Fontan surgery.

Attempts to insert prosthetic ventricular septum for single ventricle patients met with problems, leading to abandoning such procedures. Thereafter, Fontan became a preferred treatment method. With reasonably good results of Fontan, the pendulum swung so that any patient who could not undergo complete repair became a candidate for Fontan.

A middle of the road method, the so-called one-and-one-half ventricle repair was developed for patients with pulmonary atresia with intact ventricular septum with modest-sized right ventricle. In this procedure, a bidirectional Glenn procedure to divert the SVC flow into the PA is performed and allows the small right ventricle to pump the IVC blood into the pulmonary circuit, and the patent foramen ovale is closed. It is generally considered to be a better option than Fontan, although, to my knowledge, there are no comparative studies to assess this issue.

Because of relatively high mortality rates (17.0–31.7%) [39, 40] and low actuarial survival rates (66.5% at 5 years and 64.4% at 15 years) [41] for unbalanced AVSD patients following Fontan, a number of institutions attempted single stage or staged biventricular repair or conversion from single ventricle (Fontan) to biventricular repair [39, 42–47]. Detailed analysis by Nathan et al. [39] suggested that the biventricular repair and conversion from single ventricle (Fontan) to biventricular repair groups had reasonably similar mortality rates and a similar need for cardiac transplantation, but these parameters were lower than those seen in the Fontan palliation cohort.

Cardiac transplantation is a surgical alternative in the management of HLHS [48] and other single ventricle lesions. While heart transplantation was used at several institutions initially for HLHS, because of non-availability of donor hearts, most institutions have reverted to the Norwood/Fontan route. In addition, following successful cardiac transplantation, multiple medications for the prevention of graft rejection, frequent outpatient visits and periodic endomyocardial biopsy, to recognize rejection very early, are necessary in the management of these children. At the present time, cardiac transplantation is used for patients failing Fontan operation at a limited number of institutions.

4. Current status of Fontan operation

As reviewed above, since the original description in the early 1970s, the Fontan procedure has undergone numerous modifications, and, at the present time it is best described as staged total cavopulmonary connection (TCPC) with an extra-cardiac conduit and fenestration. It is performed in three stages.

4.1 Stage I

The majority, if not all, of patients who require Fontan operation (see Section 3. Indications for Fontan Operation) present during the neonatal and early infancy period, and the Fontan cannot be performed at that time because of naturally high PA pressure and high pulmonary vascular resistance (PVR). Therefore, Fontan, by necessity, becomes a multistage procedure. These babies should receive palliative intervention to allow them to reach the age and size to undergo successful Fontan surgery. The type of palliation is largely dependent upon the hemodynamic disturbance produced by multiple defects associated with a given congenital heart defect (CHD).

4.1.1 Decreased pulmonary blood flow

In neonates with decreased pulmonary blood flow, the ductus arteriosus should be kept open by administration of prostaglandin E_1 (PGE_1) intravenously at a dose of 0.05–0.1 mcg/kg/min. Once the O_2 saturation improves, the dosage of PGE_1 is gradually reduced to 0.02–0.025 mcg/kg/min to minimize the side effects of the prostaglandins. Following stabilization and diagnostic studies, as necessary to confirm the diagnosis, a more permanent way of providing pulmonary blood flow should be instituted. A number of methods to augment pulmonary blood flow have been used over the years [49, 50]. These include subclavian artery to ipsilateral PA anastomosis (classic Blalock-Taussig shunt), descending aorta to the left PA anastomosis (Potts shunt), ascending aorta to the right PA anastomosis (Waterston-Cooley shunt), SVC to right PA anastomosis, end-to-end (classic Glenn shunt), enlargement of the ventricular septal defect (VSD), formalin infiltration of the wall of the ductus arteriosus, central aortopulmonary fenestration or expanded polytetrafluoroethylene (Gore-Tex; W. L. Gore and Associates, Inc., Newark, Delaware) shunt, Gore-Tex interposition graft between the subclavian artery and the ipsilateral PA (modified Blalock-Taussig shunt), balloon pulmonary valvuloplasty, and stent implantation into the ductus arteriosus. Currently modified Blalock-Taussig (BT) shunt [51] by insertion of a Gore-Tex graft between the subclavian artery to the ipsilateral PA (**Figure 1a**) is performed by most surgeons to address pulmonary oligemia. More recently connecting the RV outflow tract with the PA via non-valve Gore-Tex graft is being used at several institutions to palliate pulmonary oligemia. Placement of a stent in the ductus arteriosus [52–54] and balloon pulmonary valvuloplasty (if the predominant obstruction is at the pulmonary valve level) [55–57] are other available options to augment the pulmonary blood flow.

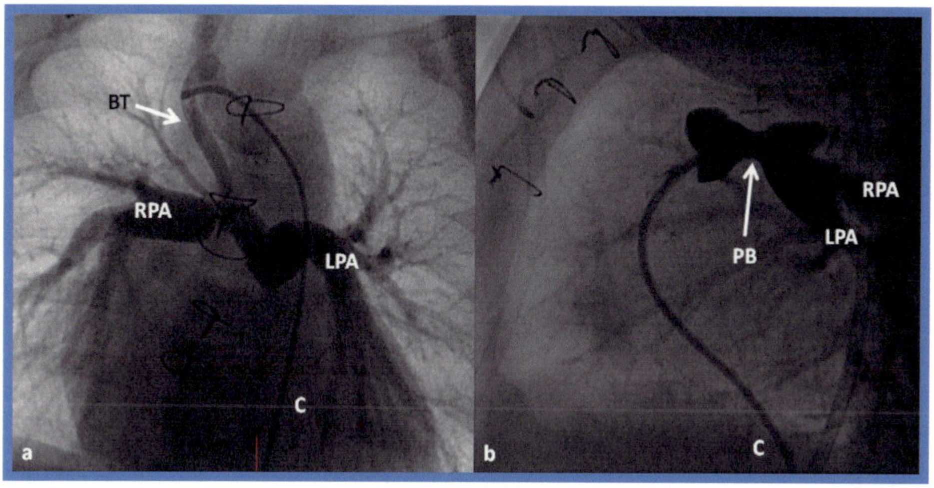

Figure 1.
Stage I Fontan. Selected frames form cineangiograms in two different babies; the first with pulmonary oligemia who received Blalock-Taussig (BT) shunt (a) and the second with pulmonary plethora who had pulmonary artery banding (PB) (b). C, catheter; LPA, left pulmonary artery; RPA, right pulmonary artery (Reproduced from [30]).

4.1.2 Increased pulmonary blood flow

In babies with increased pulmonary blood flow, optimal anti-congestive measures should be started immediately. Once the congestive heart failure (CHF) is adequately addressed, PA banding (**Figure 1b**) is performed [58] irrespective of control of CHF.

4.1.3 Normal pulmonary blood flow

Infants with near normal pulmonary blood flow with O_2 saturations in the low 80s do not need intervention and are clinically followed until Stage II.

4.1.4 Hypoplastic left heart syndrome

Neonates with hypoplastic left heart syndrome usually have Norwood palliation (**Figure 2**) [37, 59] in the neonatal period; in this operation, the following procedures are performed: (1) the main pulmonary artery and the aorta are anastomosed together; additional prosthetic material is used as needed; (2) the pulmonary circulation receives blood supply by connecting the aorta to the PA via a modified BT shunt [51] (**Figure 2b**); (3) atrial septum is excised to allow unhindered blood flow from the left to the atrium; and (4) ductal tissue is removed, and coarctation of the aorta, if present is repaired. Some surgeons use alternative Sano shunt [60], connecting the RV outflow tract to the PA (**Figure 2c**) instead of BT shunt.

4.1.5 Address other defects during Stage I

In patients with inter-atrial obstruction, it should be relieved either by transcatheter methodology or by surgery as deemed appropriate for a given clinical scenario. If there is associated coarctation of the aorta, it should also be relieved. Some patients with double-inlet left ventricle may have significant obstruction at the level of bulboventricular foramen [61]. Similarly some babies with tricuspid

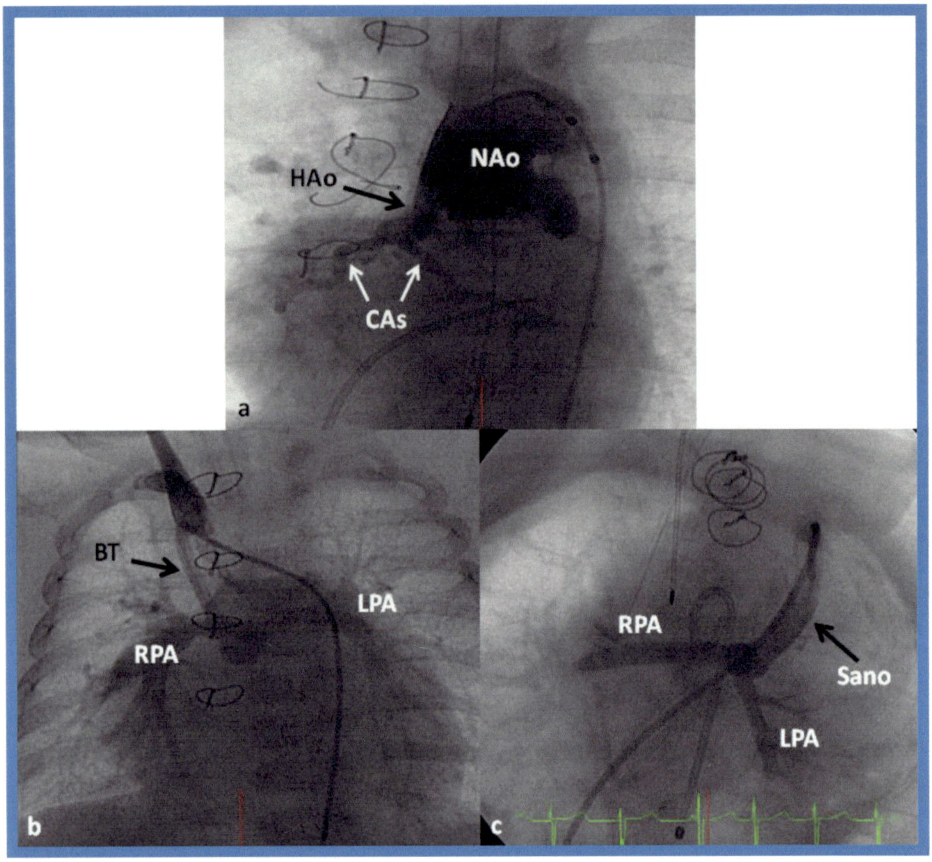

Figure 2.
Stage I Fontan for hypoplastic left heart syndrome. Selected frames from cineangiograms demonstrating Norwood operation in which the neoaorta (NAo) and hypoplastic aorta (HAo) perfuse the coronary arteries (CAs) as shown in (a), Blalock-Taussig (BT) shunt as illustrated in (b) and Sano shunt as depicted in (c). (b) and (c) are from two different babies. LPA, left pulmonary artery; RPA, right pulmonary artery (Reproduced from [30]).

atresia with transposition of the great arteries may have obstruction at the VSD level, causing obstruction to systemic blood flow [61, 62]. Such babies require Damus-Kaye-Stansel (connection of the aorta to the PA) [63] along with a BT shunt. Inter-atrial obstruction may be present frequently in babies with mitral atresia and single ventricle [64]. In such babies, predictable fall in PVR occurs following balloon or surgical relief of inter-atrial obstruction [64]; consequently, PA banding should be undertaken without hesitation at the time of relieving the atrial septal obstruction, so as to reduce the probability for CHF, lower the PVR and PA pressure, prevent pulmonary vascular obstructive disease (PVOD), and pave the way for Fontan approach [64].

4.2 Stage II

Irrespective of the type of palliative surgery in the neonatal period, bidirectional Glenn procedure [12–14, 17, 23], namely, anastomosis of the SVC to the right PA, end-to-side (**Figure 3**) is performed around the age of 6 months. The previously performed BT or Sano shunt is ligated at the same time. Although performing the procedure at 6 months is generally adopted, it can be performed as early as 3 months provided normalcy of PA pressure and anatomy can be documented.

In patients with persistent left SVC, bilateral bidirectional Glenn (**Figure 4**) is undertaken especially in patients with a small or absent left innominate vein. A bidirectional Glenn procedure may also be performed for patients with infrahepatic interruption of the IVC with azygos or hemiazygos continuation, and such a procedure is called a Kawashima procedure by some authorities.

Prior to the bidirectional Glenn procedure, normal PA pressures and adequate size of the branch PAs should be ensured by cardiac catheterization and

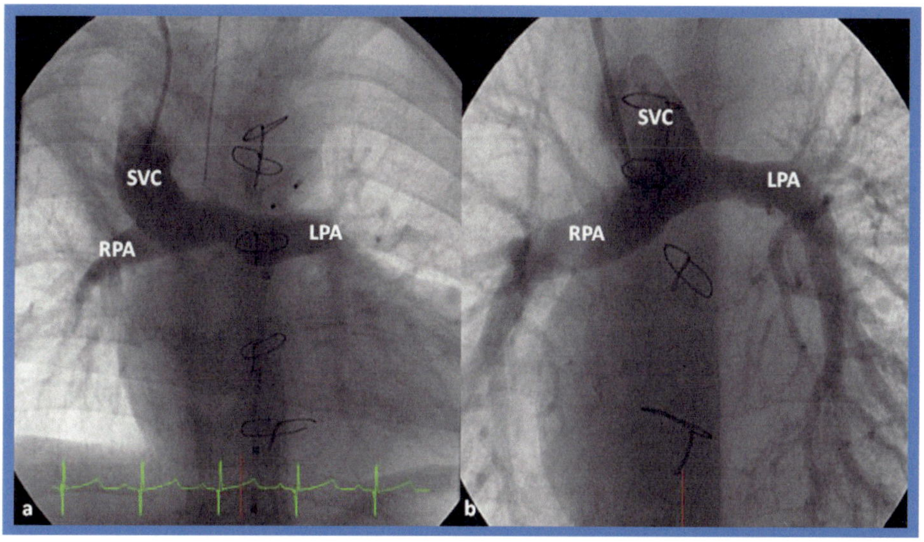

Figure 3.
Stage II of Fontan. Selected frames from cineangiograms in two different children illustrating bidirectional Glenn operation in which the superior vena cava is anastomosed to the right pulmonary artery (RPA). Unobstructed flow from the SVC to the right (RPA) and left (LPA) pulmonary arteries is clearly seen. (Reproduced from [30]).

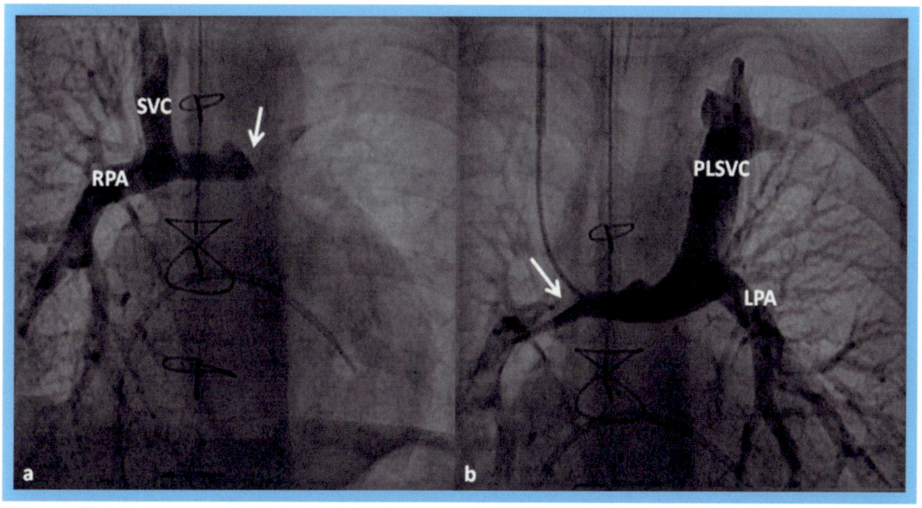

Figure 4.
Stage II Fontan. Selected frames from cineangiograms in a different child than shown in ***Figure 3****, illustrating bilateral bidirectional Glenn operation. (a) Superior vena caval angiogram demonstrates immediate visualization of the right pulmonary artery (RPA). Un-opacified blood flow from persistent left SVC (PLSVC) is indicated by the arrow in (a). (b) PLSVC angiogram illustrates rapid opacification of the left pulmonary artery (LPA). Un-opacified blood from the right SVC is shown by the arrow in (b). Flow from the respective SVCs into the pulmonary arteries is clearly seen (Reproduced from [30]).*

cineangiography. Echo-Doppler or other imaging studies (magnetic resonance imaging [MRI] or computed tomography [CT]) is advocated at some institutions.

If PA stenosis is present, it may be addressed with balloon angioplasty or stent implantation, as deemed appropriate, or it may be addressed during the bidirectional Glenn procedure. Atrioventricular valve regurgitation, aortic coarctation, subaortic obstruction, and other abnormalities should also be repaired/addressed at the time of this operation.

4.3 Stage III

During the final Stage III, the IVC flow is diverted into the PA along with creation of a fenestration. We arbitrarily divided [30] these procedures into Stage IIIA (diversion of IVC into the PA) and Stage IIIB (closure of the fenestration).

4.3.1 Stage IIIA

In the final Stage III, the total cavopulmonary connection is achieved by diverting the IVC flow into the PA either by a lateral tunnel [18, 65] or by an extra-cardiac, non-valved conduit (**Figures 5** and **6**) [21, 22]; the procedure is usually performed between the ages of 1 and 2 years, usually 1 year following the bidirectional Glenn procedure. Most surgeons seem to prefer extra-cardiac conduit to accomplish this final stage of Fontan. The majority of surgeons construct a fenestration, 4–6 mm in size, between the conduit and the atria (**Figures 5** and **6**) [27]. While the creation of fenestration during the Fontan operation was initially proposed for high-risk patients [27, 28], most surgeons now seem to prefer fenestration, since fenestration during the Fontan improves mortality rate and reduces morbidity during the immediate postoperative period [30].

Cardiac catheterization and selective cineangiography are usually performed shortly prior to Fontan conversion in order to assess the PA anatomy and pressures, trans-pulmonary gradient, PVR, and ventricular end-diastolic pressure and

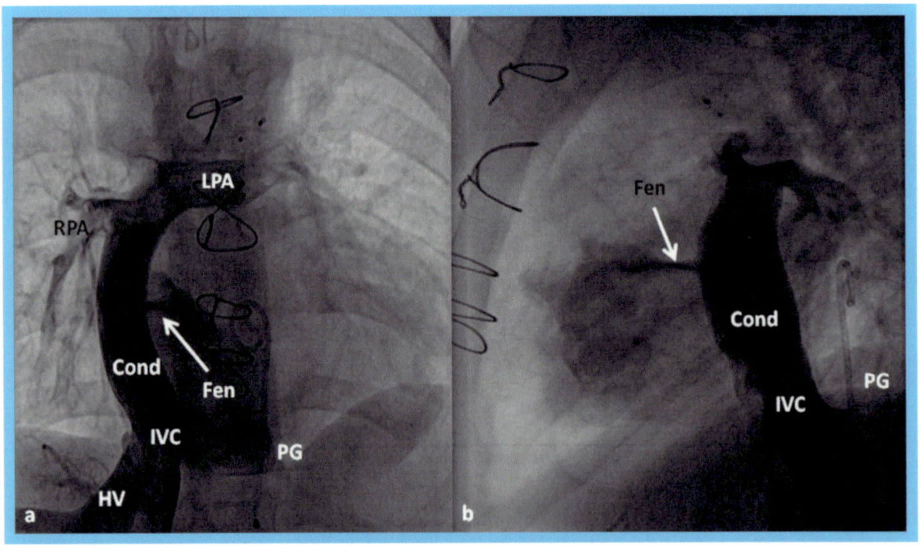

Figure 5.
Selected cine frames in posteroanterior (a) and lateral (b) views, demonstrating Stage IIIA Fontan procedure diverting the inferior vena caval flow into the pulmonary arteries via a non-valve conduit (Cond). Flow across the fenestration (fen) is shown by arrows in (a) and (b). HV, hepatic veins; LPA, left pulmonary artery; PG, pigtail catheter in the descending aorta; RPA, right pulmonary artery.

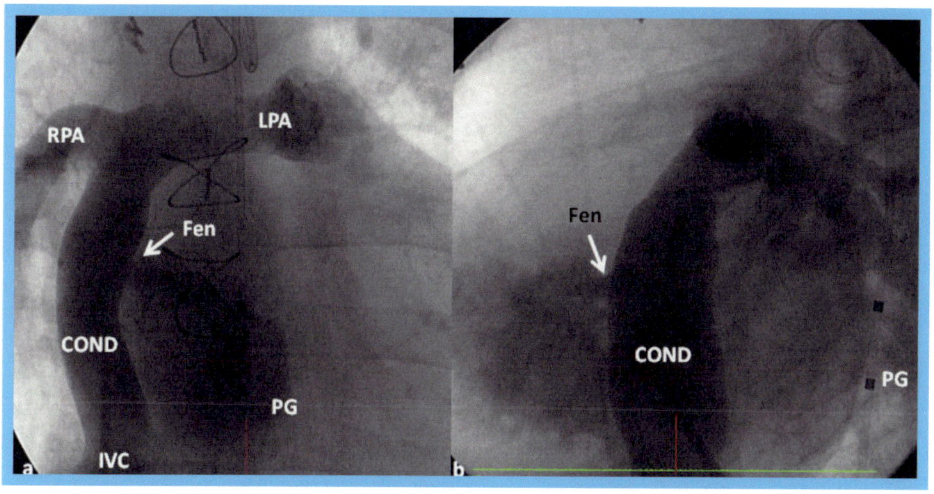

Figure 6.
Selected cine frames in posteroanterior (a) and lateral (b) views in a different patient to the one shown in ***Figure** 5, demonstrating Stage IIIA Fontan procedure diverting the inferior vena caval (IVC) flow into the pulmonary arteries via a non-valve conduit (Cond). Flow across the fenestration (fen) is shown by arrows in (a) and (b). Abbreviations are the same as those in* ***Figure** 5.*

to assure that they are normal prior to proceeding with Fontan completion. At some institutions, MRI is used for this assessment instead of catheterization and angiography; however, the author's preference is catheterization. During this catheterization, any significant collateral vessels that are present are also transcatheter-occluded by most cardiologists.

4.3.2 Stage IIIB

In the final stage, Stage IIIB, the fenestration is closed (**Figures 7b**, **8b**, and **9B** and **C**) by transcatheter methodology [27, 30–35], usually 6–12 months after Fontan Stage, IIIA. In the past, most devices used to occlude ASDs [32–35] were employed for this purpose, but at the present time, Amplatzer septal occluders are the most commonly used devices to accomplish such closures. If there are any other residual shunts, they should also be occluded (**Figure 10**) by device closure.

4.4 Interstage problems

In children who have one functioning ventricle requiring Fontan correction, the systemic and pulmonary circulations work in-parallel in place of the usual in-series circulation. A fragile equilibrium between the two circulations must be preserved so that adequate systemic and pulmonary perfusions are maintained. There is substantial interstage mortality ranging from 5 to 15% [66–68] which may be due to restrictive atrial communication, obstruction of the aortic arch, blockage of the shunt, distortion of the PAs, atrioventricular valve insufficiency, or a combination thereof [66]. Intercurrent illnesses such as dehydration, respiratory tract illness, or fever disturb this balance and make the patients to become critically ill and have been blamed for interstage mortality [66, 68]. The surgically created BT and Sano shunts may also get thrombosed producing severe hypoxemia [69]. Indeed, these abnormalities produce significant interstage mortality [67]; these appear to occur more frequently between Stages I and II than between Stages II and III. Consequently, extreme vigilance in managing these patients should be maintained by the caregiver [68, 70]; even trivial illnesses must be aggressively monitored and addressed as appropriate.

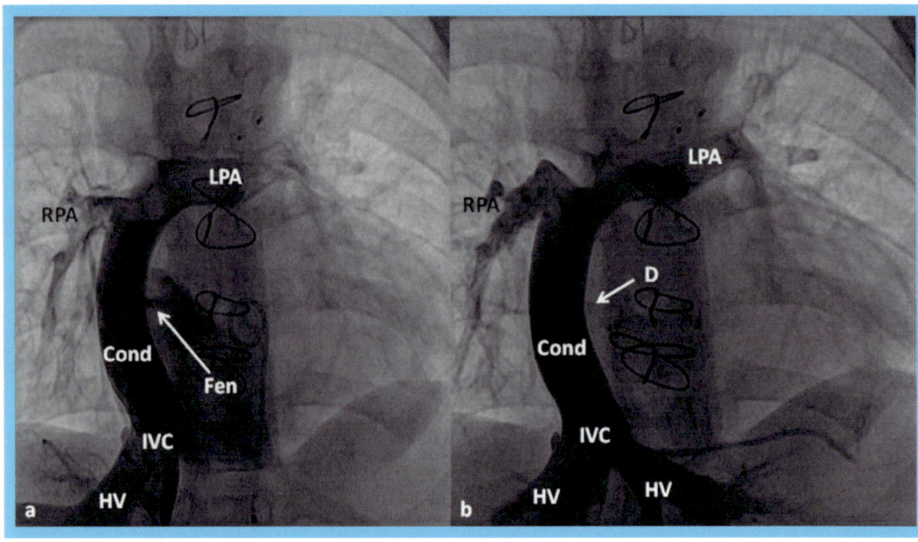

Figure 7.
Stage IIIB. (a) Selected frames from cineangiograms in anteroposterior projection illustrating Stage IIIA of the Fontan operation in which the inferior vena caval (IVC) flow is diverted into the pulmonary arteries by a non-valve conduit (Cond). The fenestration (fen) is shown by the arrow in (a). (b) Closure of the fenestration with an Amplatzer septal occluder device (D) is shown with an arrow in (b). HV, hepatic veins; LPA, left pulmonary artery; RPA, right pulmonary artery (Reproduced from [30]).

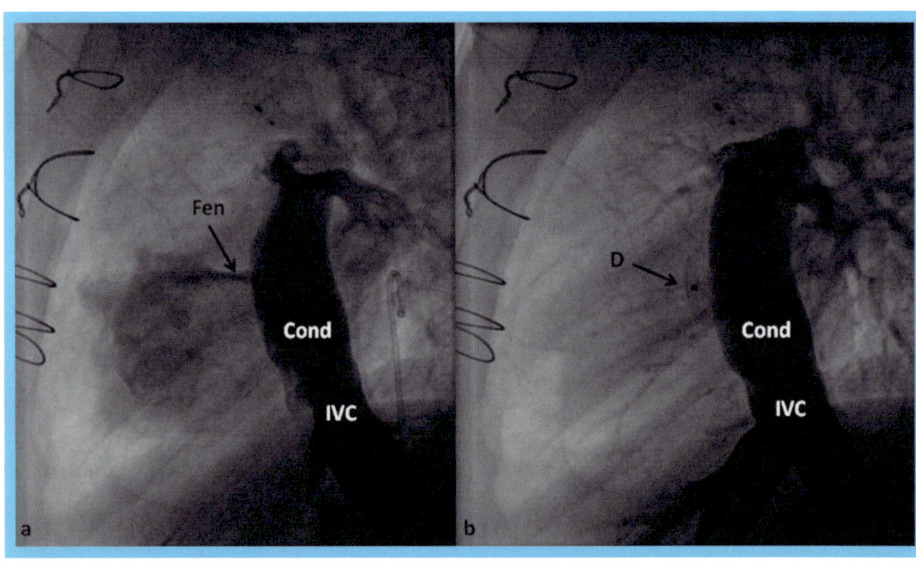

Figure 8.
Stage IIIB. (a) Selected frames from cineangiograms in lateral view of the same patient illustrated in **Figure 5** *showing Stage IIIA of the Fontan operation in which the inferior vena caval (IVC) flow is diverted into the pulmonary arteries by a non-valve conduit (Cond). The fenestration (fen) is shown by the arrow in (a). (b) Closure of the fenestration with an Amplatzer septal occluder device (D) is shown with an arrow in (b). (Stage IIIB). Reproduced from [30].*

5. Results of Fontan operation

Immediate and follow-up results of both older and current types of Fontan will be reviewed in this section.

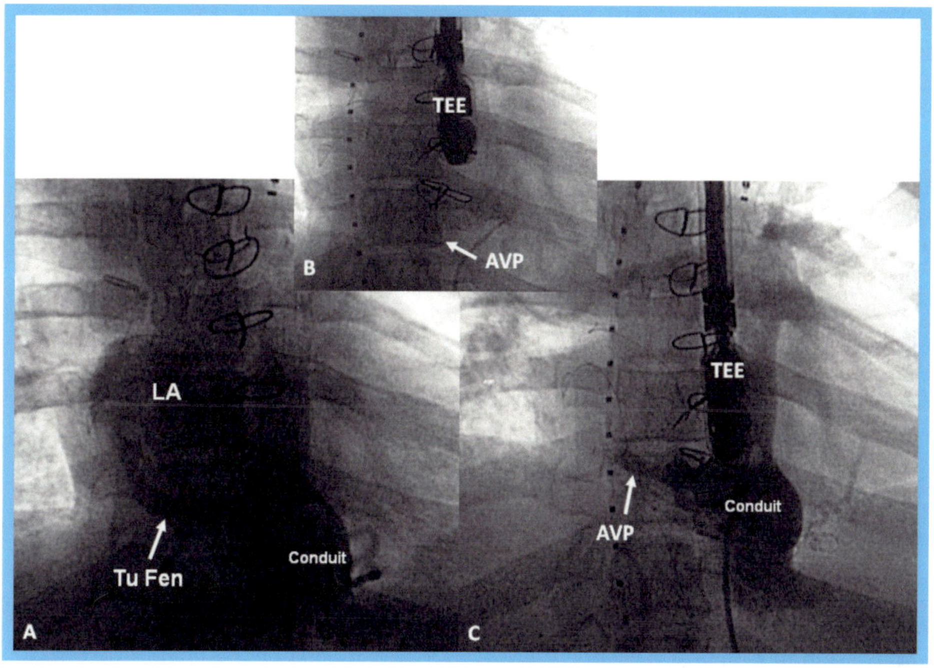

Figure 9.
(A) Selected cine frame from a Fontan conduit cineangiogram in anteroposterior view, demonstrating tubular fenestration (Tu fen) with opacification of the left atrium (LA). (B) The Tu fen is closed with an Amplatzer vascular plug (AVP). (C) A follow-up conduit cineangiogram after AVP implantation, showing complete occlusion of the Tu fen. TEE, transesophageal probe.

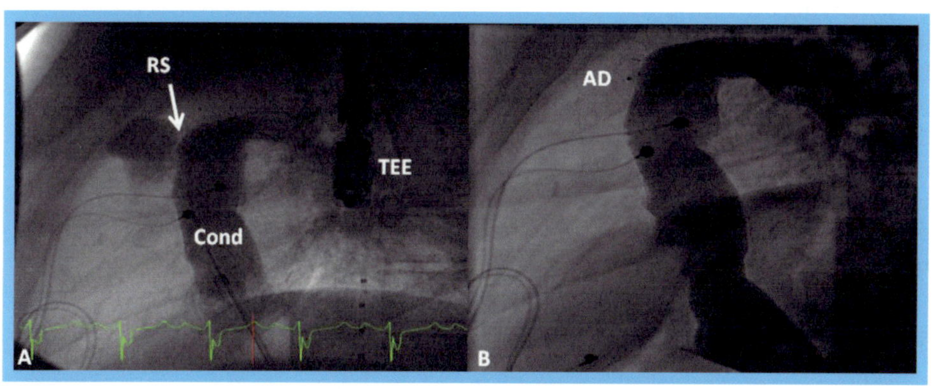

Figure 10.
(A) A selected cineangiographic frame showing the Fontan conduit in lateral view, demonstrating a residual shunt (RS) at the superior aspect of the conduit (Cond). (B) The RS was occluded with an Amplatzer septal occluder device (AD); the residual shunt is no longer seen. TEE, transesophageal echo probe.

5.1 Immediate results

The results of original Fontan [1, 2] and its earlier modifications, namely, RA-to-PA or RA-to-RV anastomosis either directly or via valved or non-valved conduits, revealed high initial mortality rates. The initial mortality rates ranged from 10 to 26% [9, 10, 71, 72]. Furthermore, the postoperative stay in the intensive care setting was prolonged.

The initial mortality following staged, total cavopulmonary connection has decreased remarkably [73–78]. Patients who had total cavopulmonary connection without fenestration had initial mortality rates ranging from 8 to 10.5% [73–75], while subjects who had total cavopulmonary connection with fenestration had slightly lower (4.5–7.5%) initial mortality rates [76–78].

In one large single institutional study examining the results of 500 consecutive Fontan surgery patients [77], early failure was associated with high (≥19 mm Hg) mean PA pressure, young age at surgery, heterotaxy syndrome, a right-sided tricuspid valve as systemic atrioventricular valve, distorted pulmonary arteries, an atriopulmonary connection, no Fontan fenestration, and longer cardiopulmonary bypass time.

These investigators also observed that a significant improvement in morbidity and mortality from early (first quartile—early failures: 27.1%) to the more recent time (last quartile—early failures: 7.5%) occurred [77]. This progress appears to be related to increasing surgical and intensive care experience as well as to more recently introduced Fontan modifications.

5.2 Follow-up results

Long-term follow-up results were also poor with older types of Fontan [9, 10]. The late mortality rates varied from 1 to 11%, and when early and late mortality rates were combined, they varied between 11 and 25%. The need for reoperations was present in 1–11% of patients. Factors adversely influencing late mortality and reoperation rates are earlier calendar year of operation, age of patient at the time of surgery, type of prior palliative procedures, hypoplasia, distortion or obstruction of PAs, subaortic obstruction, significant mitral valve insufficiency, elevated PA pressure or resistance, decreased left ventricular function, increased left ventricular muscle mass, asplenia syndrome, and others [9, 10].

Following the introduction of staged cavopulmonary anastomosis (both lateral tunnel and extra-cardiac conduit diversion of IVC blood to the PA), the long-term outcomes have improved. In one study in which results of follow-up for 10.2 ± 0.6 years of 196 patients were examined, the estimated Kaplan-Meier survival was 93 and 91% at 5 and 10 years, respectively [79]. An equally impressive finding was freedom from supraventricular arrhythmias in 96 and 91% of patients at 5 and 10 years following surgery. In a different study, the actuarial survival 15 years following surgery was 85% [80]. But, late re-interventions were necessary in 12.7% of patients. When lateral tunnel and extra-cardiac conduit types of Fontan were compared, the outcomes were found to be similar for both groups [81, 82].

Using fenestration during Fontan appears to improve early mortality and morbidity, particularly demonstrated in high-risk patents [83]. A more recent analysis in a smaller group of patients did not demonstrate significant advantage of fenestrated Fontan over the non-fenestrated [84]. However, the general consensus is that using fenestration during Fontan decreases mortality and morbidity during the postoperative period [30, 76–78].

6. Follow-up protocol and complications

Periodic follow-up following Fontan is generally recommended. These patients are evaluated at 1, 6, and 12 months after Stage IIIB (device closure of fenestration) and yearly thereafter. During the follow-up, platelet-inhibiting doses of aspirin 2–5 mg/kg/day in children or clopidogrel 75 mg/day in adults to prevent thrombus formation and angiotensin-converting enzyme inhibitors for afterload reduction are generally prescribed. Electrocardiograms and echocardiograms are generally performed during evaluation of these patients with additional imaging studies, as indicated. Any abnormalities, as and when detected, are addressed.

During follow-up, a number of complications were reported, and these include arrhythmias, obstructed Fontan pathways, cyanosis, paradoxical emboli, thrombi, development of collateral vessels, and protein loosing enteropathy [30, 31, 85]. These complications appear to be more frequent with older types of Fontan than with the currently used staged, total cavopulmonary connection with extra-cardiac conduit and fenestration. When such complications develop, they should be promptly investigated and treated. In the ensuing paragraphs, a brief review of some of these complications will be presented.

6.1 Arrhythmias

Arrhythmias were more frequently seen in patients with old Fontan (atriopulmonary connection) than with staged TCPC. The observed arrhythmias were typically atrial arrhythmias, namely, atrial flutter/fibrillation and supraventricular tachycardia. Initially, anti-arrhythmic medications are used to control the rhythm disturbance. This should be followed by hemodynamic and angiographic assessment to identify obstructive lesions in the Fontan pathways. The obstructive lesions should be treated with balloon angioplasty, stent, or surgery, as applicable. Continued rhythm abnormality calls for radiofrequency ablation. Although the success rate of radiofrequency ablation is high in 80% range [86], rates of recurrence range from 30 to 40%. In subjects who have resistant arrhythmias, reducing the atrial mass, switch to TCPC with concomitant Maize procedure is advisable [87]. A few patients develop atrioventricular block or sick sinus syndrome which may require pacemaker implantation. Fortunately, ventricular arrhythmias are less frequent.

6.2 Development of obstruction in Fontan pathways

Obstructions in Fontan circulation may occur. Obstructive lesions in the SVC or IVC may arise but are less frequently seen. However, branch pulmonary artery stenoses may be seen more often. Obstructions within the lateral tunnel or extra-cardiac conduit are also uncommon, but may occur due to thrombus formation and will be addressed in the section on "Thrombus formation." In the presence of signs and symptoms indicative of obstruction in the Fontan pathway, prompt investigation to confirm such obstruction should be made. While echo studies are useful in young children, poor echo windows in adolescents and adults may require MRI and CT, and/or angiographic studies to confirm or exclude such obstructive lesions. If the obstructive lesions are detected, they should be promptly relieved by balloon angioplasty or stent implantation (**Figure 11**) [88]. Surgery may be needed in rare occasions.

6.3 Residual arterial desaturation and paradoxical emboli

Sometimes connections between lateral tunnel and extra-cardiac conduit on the one hand and the atrium on the other persist. These residual defects and intentionally created Fontan fenestrations result in right-to-left shunt because the pressure in the Fontan conduit is higher than that of the atrial pressures. These residual defects will result in arterial desaturation and may become the site of paradoxical embolism with consequential transient ischemic attacks (TIAs), cerebrovascular accidents (CVAs), and systemic emboli. These residual defects as well as Fontan fenestrations should be occluded by transcatheter techniques

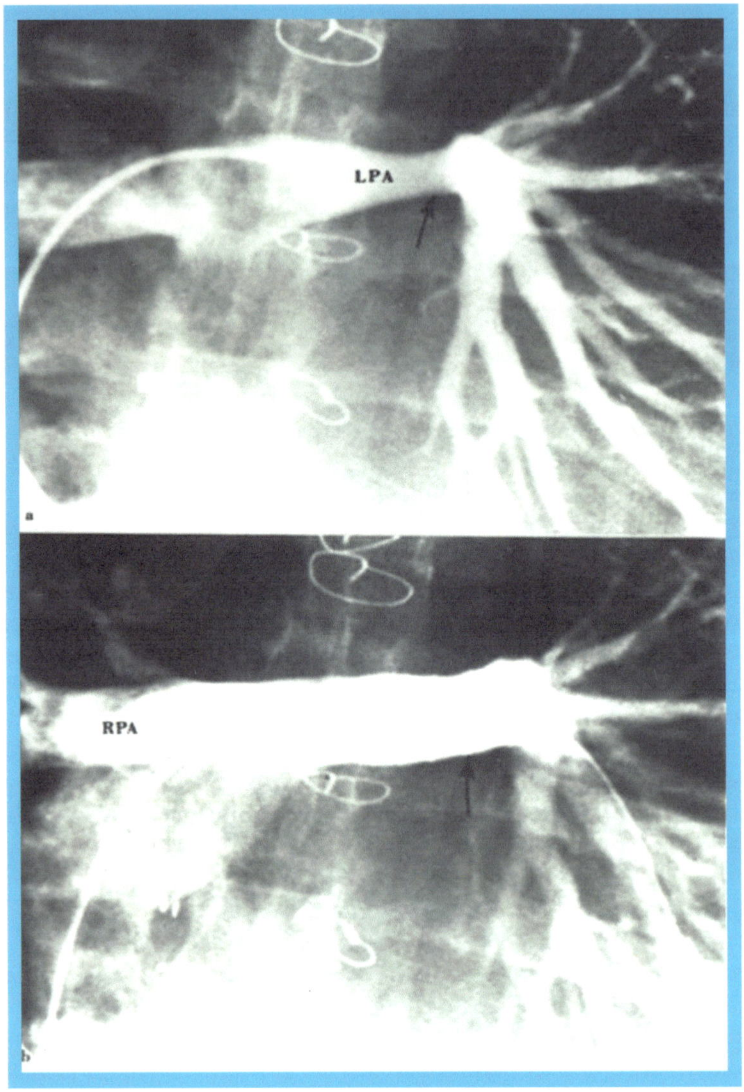

Figure 11.
Selected frames from cineangiograms of the pulmonary artery in posteroanterior view illustrating normal right pulmonary artery (RPA) and narrowed (arrow) left pulmonary artery (LPA) prior to (a) and after (b) stent (arrow) placement in an adolescent who had Fontan surgery several years earlier (Reproduced from [88]).

to return O2 saturations to normal and decrease the likelihood for paradoxical embolism [30, 32, 33, 83, 88, 89]. Amplatzer septal occluder (St. Jude Medical, Inc., St Paul, MN) is currently most common device used to accomplish this (**Figures 7**, **8**, and **10**). Tubular fenestrations may be closed with Amplatzer vascular plug devices (St. Jude Medical, Inc.) (**Figure 9**). Test occlusion of the residual defect or fenestration is suggested to ensure that adequate cardiac output is maintained following defect occlusion [89, 90], especially if the procedure is performed shortly after fenestrated Fontan. Late follow-up results of fenestration closure are good [33].

6.4 Thrombus formation

There is a tendency for thrombus formation in the Fontan pathway; the reported prevalence was 15–30% [91, 92]. Regrettably the usual transthoracic echo-Doppler evaluation may not discover these thrombi. However, transesophageal echocardiography, MRI, or CT studies may be necessary to detect these thrombi. In an attempt to prevent thrombus formation in the Fontan circuit, thromboprophylaxis is commonly recommended; both warfarin and aspirin have been utilized in the past for this purpose. A multicenter, randomized trial was conducted to compare the efficacy of these two drugs; results showed less than optimal results with both drugs and no significant difference between the two regimens [93]. In the author's experience, most children are prescribed with aspirin for thromboprophylaxis which may be switched to clopidogrel (Plavix) as the children approach adulthood.

Despite seemingly adequate thromboprophylaxis, some patients develop thrombosis of the Fontan conduits (**Figure 12A**). We initially employ thrombus dissolving drug therapy (tPA, heparin, etc.). If the thrombi do not resolve, we have employed stenting of the conduit to compress the thrombi against the conduit wall [94]. An example from our experience is shown in **Figure 12**.

6.5 Development of collateral vessels

Systemic venous to pulmonary venous and systemic arterial to pulmonary arterial collateral vessels may develop in some patients after the Fontan procedure [88, 95]. These may develop both shortly after the procedure and during late follow-up. Systemic venous to pulmonary venous collateral vessels produce arterial hypoxemia. In addition, they may also become potential sites for paradoxical embolism.

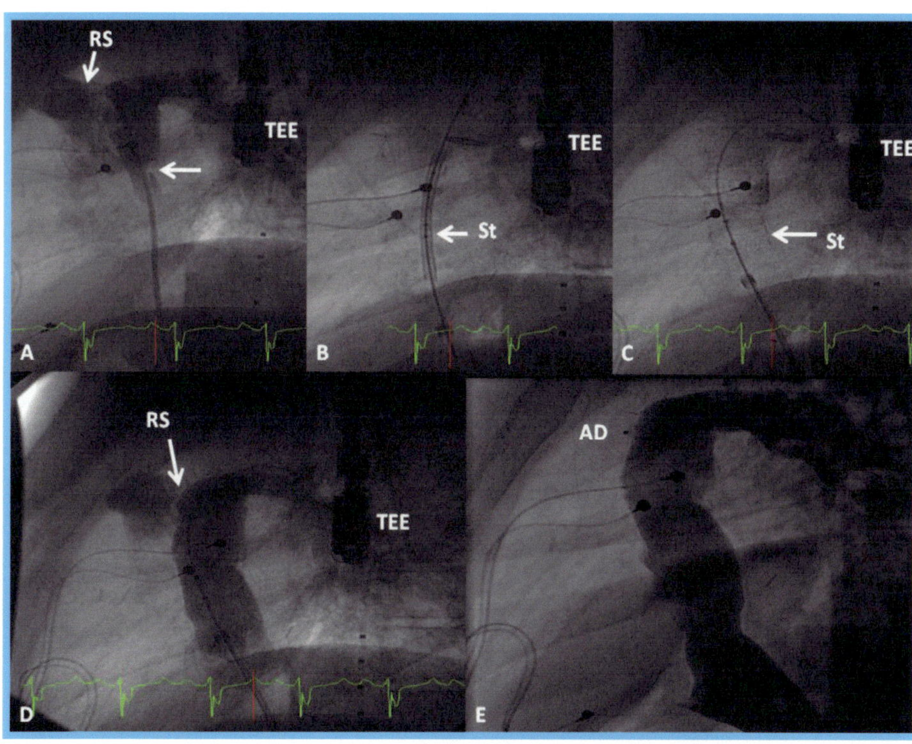

Figure 12.
(A) Selected frame from a cineangiogram of a Fontan conduit in lateral view, illustrating a thrombus (arrow in (A)). (B) and (C) position of a stent (St) before (B) and after (C) its complete expansion. (D) Cineangiographic frame demonstrating the widely patent stent after stent deployment. Also, note the residual shunt (RS) at the superior aspect of the conduit (seen in (A) and (D)). The RS was occluded with an Amplatzer septal occluder device (AD) shortly after the cine shown in (D). (F) A follow-up cineangiogram 1 year later shows the continued patency of the conduit with no RS. TEE, transesophageal echo probe (Reproduced from [94]).

Systemic arterial to pulmonary arterial (or venous) collateral vessels produce left ventricular volume overload. These abnormal vessels should be transcatheter-occluded with coils, vascular plugs, and ductal occluding devices depending upon the size and accessibility. Examples from the author's experience of occluding these vessels are shown in **Figures 13–16** [88, 95, 96].

6.6 Protein loosing enteropathy

Protein losing enteropathy (PLE) is a grave long-term complication of Fontan with a prevalence of 11.1% in older types of Fontan [85, 97]. However, the incidence appears to have come down to 1.2% with staged TCPC [85, 98]. The reason for development of PLE is not understood. Intestinal protein loss secondary to lymphatic distension which in turn may be due to elevated pressure in systemic veins is considered to be a pathogenic mechanism. But, PLE has been seen even in patients with "normal" Fontan circuit pressures. Therefore, the true cause of PLE remains a mystery. The symptoms and signs of PLE are diarrhea, edema, ascites, and/or pleural effusions. Laboratory abnormalities include reduced serum albumin and elevated fecal alpha-1 antitrypsin levels. The PLE diagnosis may be confirmed with technetium 99m-labeled human serum albumin scintigraphy [99].

Because of high mortality rate seen with PLE, speedy diagnosis and implementing aggressive management strategies are important [85]. At first, supportive therapy such as medium-chain triglycerides diet, infusion of intravenous albumin, and replacement of immunoglobulins should be undertaken. Obstructive lesions in the Fontan pathway should be scrutinized, and aortopulmonary connections should be screened for. If identified, they should be treated with appropriate transcatheter measures. Surgical therapy is indicated if they cannot be adequately addressed with transcatheter intervention. A variety of other treatment regimens, including prednisone, elementary diet, calcium replacement, regular high-molecular-weight heparin, low-molecular-weight heparin, somatostatin, high-dose spironolactone, sildenafil, and resection of localized intestinal lymphangiectasia, have been utilized in the past with varying degrees of success [85].

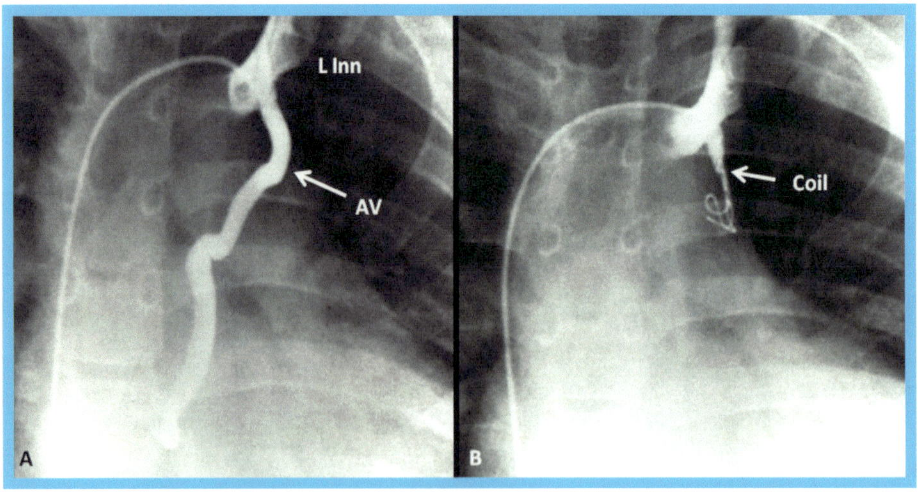

Figure 13.
(a) Selected frame from a left innominate vein (L inn) cineangiogram in posteroanterior view demonstrating an anomalous vein (AV) opacifying the atrial mass (not marked). (b) Following occlusion with Gianturco coil (arrow), the AV is completely occluded and the systemic arterial saturation improved (Reproduced from [88]).

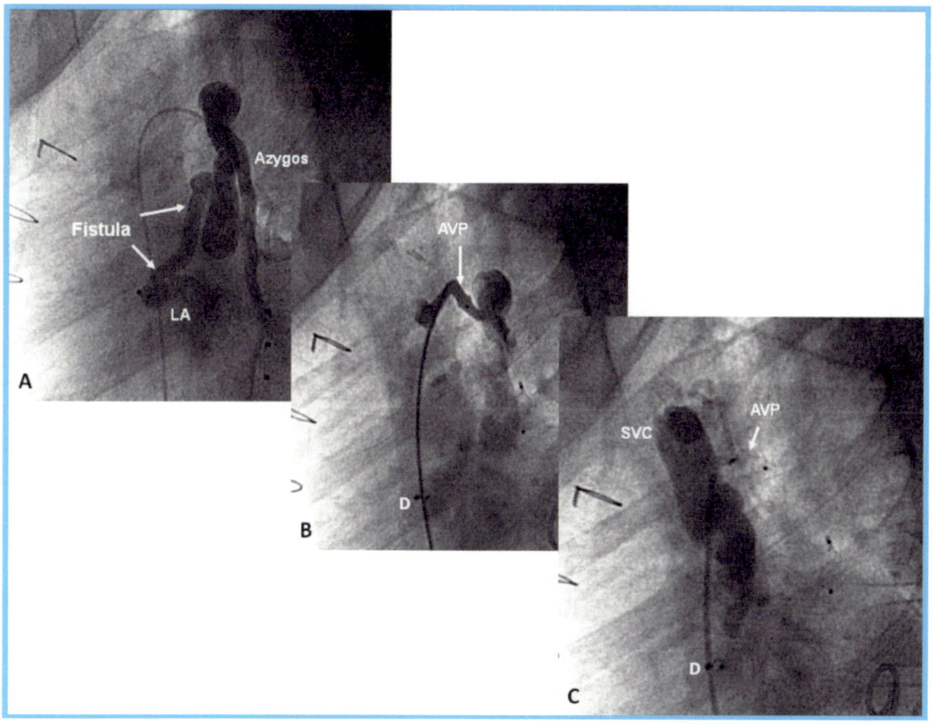

Figure 14.
(A) Selected frame from a cineangiogram in lateral view with the catheter positioned at the superior vena cava/azygos junction illustrating a fistula which results in opacification of the left atrium (LA). (B) The fistula was occluded with an Amplatzer vascular plug (arrow—AVP) with some residual flow. (C) Follow-up SVC injection shows complete occlusion by the AVP (Reproduced from [96]).

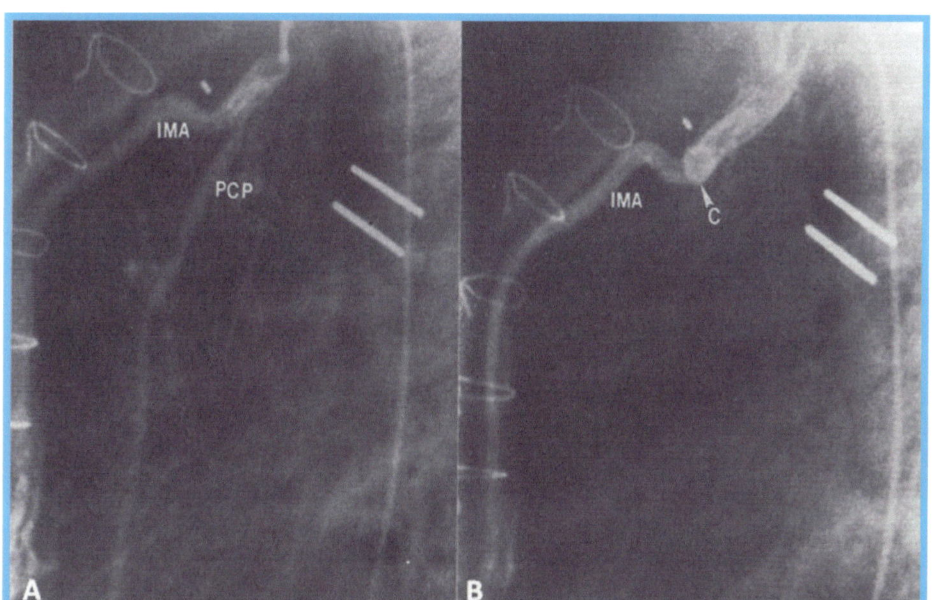

Figure 15.
(A) Selected cine frame from an internal mammary artery (IMA) cineangiogram in the lateral view, demonstrating multiple small collateral vessels arising from the pericardiophrenic (PCP) branch, which resulted in a significant levophase (not shown). (B) Following occlusion with a Gianturco coil (C), there is complete occlusion of this vessel (Reproduced from [95]).

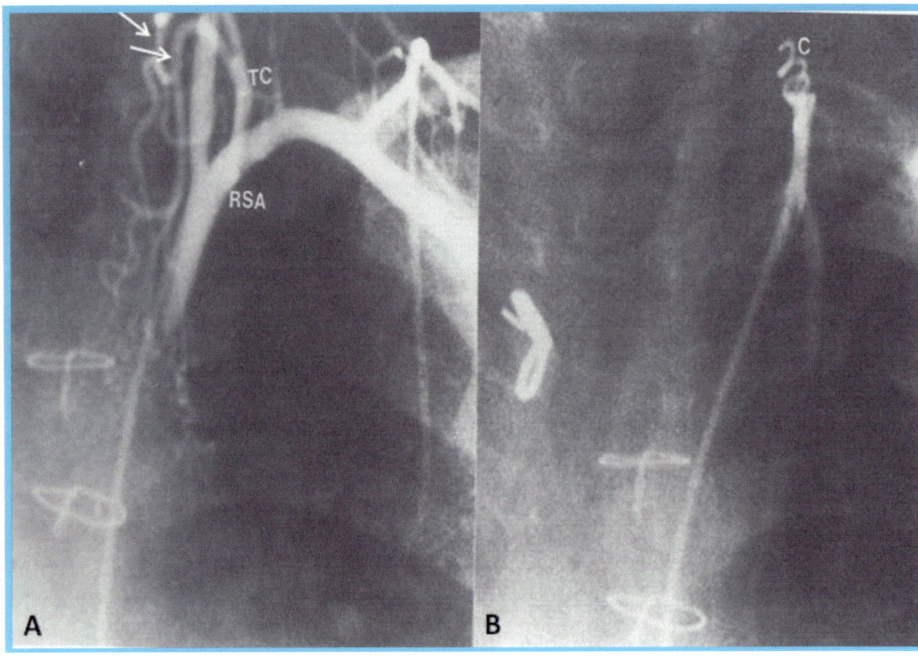

Figure 16.
(A) Selected cine frame from a right subclavian artery (RSA) cineangiogram showing branches (white arrows) of the thyrocervical (TC) trunk which supplied a number of small vessels, giving a good degree of levophase. (B) Complete occlusion occurred following the implantation of a Gianturco coil (C) (Reproduced from [95]).

Following a short trial of any of the above treatment modes, largely on the basis of the cardiologist's preference, a more definitive treatment methods such as lessening the conduit pressure by creating a fenestration between the conduit and the atrium [99–101], converting atriopulmonary type of Fontan to TCPC [87, 102, 103], instituting sequential atrioventricular pacing [104, 105], and performing cardiac transplantation [106–108] should all be considered. Again, it is essential to emphasize that timely treatment should be instituted as soon as PLE is identified [85]. Fortunately, the need for use of these methods has progressively diminished since the wide use of staged TCPC.

7. Summary and conclusions

Since the initial description of the Fontan operation in the early 1970s by Fontan, Kruetzer, and their associates, several modifications have been introduced. These include avoiding classic Glenn anastomosis; not using a prosthetic valve in the IVC; RA-PA anastomosis, direct or through a non-valved conduit; RA-PA anastomosis through a valved conduit; RA-RV anastomosis, direct or non-valved anastomosis; RA-RV anastomosis through a valved conduit; bidirectional Glenn procedure (cavopulmonary anastomosis); lateral tunnel; total cavopulmonary connection; extra-cardiac conduit, staged Fontan; fenestrated Fontan; and closure of Fontan fenestration. Currently staged, total cavopulmonary connection with extra-cardiac conduit and fenestration has become the most commonly used multistage surgery in accomplishing the Fontan.

The indications for Fontan are patients who have one functioning ventricle, and these include tricuspid atresia, double-inlet left ventricle, HLHS, mitral atresia with normal aortic root, unbalanced AVSDs, pulmonary atresia with intact ventricular septum with markedly hypoplastic right ventricle, and other complex heart defects with one functioning ventricle. Recently there has been a trend for biventricular repair, particularly for patients with unbalanced AVSDs.

Stage I consists of performing palliative procedures on the basis of pathophysiology of the defect complex at presentation, usually in the neonatal period. Stage II involves performing a bidirectional Glenn procedure (diversion of the superior vena caval blood flow into both lungs) usually at about the age of 6 months. During stage IIIA diversion of the IVC blood flow into the lungs, usually by an extra-cardiac conduit plus a fenestration, usually at about the age of 2 years. Stage IIIB consists of transcatheter closure of the fenestration 6–12 months after Stage IIIA.

Both the immediate and follow-up results have remarkably improved, both in terms of mortality and morbidity, following the introduction of staged total cavo-pulmonary connection with extra-cardiac conduit and fenestration with subsequent catheter closure of Fontan fenestration. Complications do occur during follow-up, and they should be addressed as and when they are detected.

Conflict of interest

The author declares no conflict of interest.

Author details

P. Syamasundar Rao
University of Texas at Houston, McGovern Medical School and Children's Memorial Hermann Hospital, Houston, TX, USA

*Address all correspondence to: p.syamasundar.rao@uth.tmc.edu

References

[1] Fontan F, Baudet E. Surgical repair of tricuspid atresia. Thorax. 1971;**26**:240-248

[2] Kreutzer G, Bono H, Galindez E. Una operacion para la correccion de la atresia tricuspidea. In: Ninth Argent Congress of Cardiology; Buenos Aires, Argentina; 1971

[3] Glenn WW. Circulatory bypass of the right side of the heart. IV. Shunt between superior vena cava and distal right pulmonary artery; report of clinical application. The New England Journal of Medicine. 1958;**259**:117-120

[4] Rao PS. Tricuspid Atresia. Mount Kisco: Futura Publishing Co.; 1982

[5] Rao PS. Tricuspid Atresia. 2nd ed. Mt Kisco: Futura Publishing Co.; 1992

[6] Rao PS. Tricuspid atresia. In: Moller JH, Hoffman JIE, editors. Pediatric Cardiovascular Medicine. New York: Churchill Livingstone; 2000. pp. 421-441

[7] Rao PS. Tricuspid atresia. In: Moller JH, Hoffman JIE, editors. Pediatric Cardiovascular Medicine. 2nd ed. Oxford: Wiley-Blackwell/A John Wiley & Sons Ltd.; 2012. pp. 487-508

[8] Rao PS. Tricuspid atresia. In: Vijayalakshmi IB, Rao PS, Chugh R, editors. A Comprehensive Approach to Management of Congenital Heart Diseases. New Delhi: Jaypee Publications; 2013. pp. 397-413

[9] Chopra PS, Rao PS. Corrective surgery for tricuspid atresia: Which modification of Fontan-Kreutzer procedure should be used? A review. American Heart Journal. 1992;**123**:758-767

[10] Rao PS, Chopra PS. Modifications of Fontan-Kreutzer procedure for tricuspid atresia: Can a choice be made? In: Rao PS, editor. Tricuspid Atresia. 2nd ed. Mount Kisco, New York: Futura; 1992. pp. 361-375

[11] Haller JA Jr, Adkins JC, Worthington M, Rauenhorst J. Experimental studies on permanent bypass of the right heart. Surgery. 1966;**59**:1128-1132

[12] Azzolina G, Eufrate S, Pensa P. Tricuspid atresia: Experience in surgical management with a modified cavopulmonary anastomosis. Thorax. 1972;**27**:111-115

[13] Kawashima Y, Kitamura S, Matsuda H, Shimazaki Y, Nakano S, Hirose H. Total cavopulmonary shunt operation in complex cardiac anomalies. The Journal of Thoracic and Cardiovascular Surgery. 1984;**87**:74-81

[14] Hopkins RA, Armstrong SE, Serwer GA, Peterson RJ, Old-ham HN. Physiologic rationale for a bidirectional cavopulmonary shunt: A versatile complement to the Fontan principle. The Journal of Thoracic and Cardiovascular Surgery. 1985;**90**:391-398

[15] DiDonato R, DiCarlo DC, Giannico S, Marcelletti C. Palliation of complex cardiac anomalies with subaortic obstruction: New operative approach. Journal of the American College of Cardiology. 1989;**13**:406-412

[16] Mazzera E, Corno A, Picardo S, et al. Bidirectional cavopulmonary shunts: Clinical applications as staged or definitive palliation. The Annals of Thoracic Surgery. 1989;**47**:415-420

[17] Bridges ND, Jonas RA, Mayer JE, Flanagan MF, Keane JF, Castaneda AR. Bidirectional cavopulmonary anastomosis as interim palliation for high-risk Fontan

candidates: Early results. Circulation. 1990;**82**(Suppl IV):170-176

[18] Puga FJ, Chiavarelli M, Hagler DJ, et al. Circulation. 1987;**76**(Suppl III):III-53-III-60

[19] de Leval MR, Kilner P, Gewillig M, Bull C. Total cavopulmonary connection: A logical alternative to atriopulmonary connection for complex Fontan operations. Experimental studies and early clinical experience. The Journal of Thoracic and Cardiovascular Surgery. 1988;**96**:682-695

[20] Sharma S, Goudy S, Walker P, et al. In vitro flow experiments for determination of optimal geometry of total cavopulmonary connection for surgical repair of children with functional single ventricle. Journal of the American College of Cardiology. 1996;**27**:1264-1269

[21] Marcelletti C, Corno A, Giannico S, Marino B. Inferior vena cava-pulmonary artery extra-cardiac conduit. A new form of right heart bypass. The Journal of Thoracic and Cardiovascular Surgery. 1990;**100**:228-232

[22] Marcelletti C, Iorio FS, Abella RF. Late results of extra-cardiac Fontan repair. Seminars in Thoracic and Cardiovascular Surgery: Pediatric Cardiac Surgery Annual. 1999;**2**:131-141

[23] Pridjian AK, Mendelsohn AM, Lupinetti FM, et al. Usefulness of the bidirectional Glenn procedure as staged reconstruction for the functional single ventricle. The American Journal of Cardiology. 1993;**71**:959-962

[24] Norwood WI, Jacobs ML. Fontan's procedure in two stages. American Journal of Surgery. 1993;**166**:548-551

[25] Choussat A, Fontan F, Besse P, et al. Selection criteria for Fontan procedure. In: Anderson RH, Shinebourne EA, editors. Pediatric Cardiology. White Plains, NY: Churchill Livingstone; 1978. p. 559

[26] Billingsley AM, Laks H, Boyce SW, George B, Santulli T, Williams RG. Definitive repair in patients with pulmonary atresia and intact ventricular septum. The Journal of Thoracic and Cardiovascular Surgery. 1989;**97**:746-754

[27] Bridges ND, Lock JE, Castaneda AR. Baffle fenestration with subsequent transcatheter closure. Modification of the Fontan operation for patients at increased risk. Circulation. 1990;**82**:1681-1689

[28] Laks H, Pearl JM, Haas GS, et al. Partial Fontan: Advantages of an adjustable interatrial communication. The Annals of Thoracic Surgery. 1991;**52**:1084-1094; discussion 1094-1095

[29] Thompson LD, Petrossian E, McElhinney DB, et al. Is it necessary to routinely fenestrate an extra-cardiac Fontan? Journal of the American College of Cardiology. 1999;**34**:539-544

[30] Rao PS. Fontan operation: Indications, short and long term outcomes. Indian Journal of Pediatrics. 2015;**82**:1147-1156

[31] Rao PS. Pediatric tricuspid atresia. Medscape Drugs & Diseases. 2016. Available from: http://emedicine.medscape.com/article/900832-overview

[32] Rao PS, Chandar JS, Sideris EB. Role of inverted buttoned device in transcatheter occlusion of atrial septal defects or patent foramen ovale with right-to-left shunting associated with previously operated complex congenital cardiac anomalies. The American Journal of Cardiology. 1997;**80**:914-921

[33] Goff DA, Blume ED, Gauvreau K, Mayer JE, Lock JE, Jenkins KJ. Clinical

outcome of fenestrated Fontan patients after closure: The first 10 years. Circulation. 2000;**102**:2094-2099

[34] Boudjemline Y, Bonnet D, Sidi D, Agnoletti G. Closure of extrocardiac Fontan fenestration by using the Amplatzer duct occluder. Archives des Maladies du Coeur et des Vaisseaux. 2005;**98**:449-454

[35] Rothman A, Evans WN, Mayman GA. Percutaneous fenestration closure with problematic residual native atrial septum. Catheterization and Cardiovascular Interventions. 2005;**66**:286-290

[36] Gale AW, Danielson GK, McGoon DC, Mair DD. Modified Fontan operation for univentricular heart and complicated congenital lesions. The Journal of Thoracic and Cardiovascular Surgery. 1979;**78**:831-838

[37] Norwood WI, Lang P, Castaneda AR, et al. Experience with operation for hypoplastic left heart syndrome. The Journal of Thoracic and Cardiovascular Surgery. 1981;**82**:511-519

[38] Norwood WI, Lang P, Hansen DD. Physiologic repair of aortic atresia-hypoplastic left heart syndrome. The New England Journal of Medicine. 1983;**308**:23-26

[39] Nathan M, Emani S, Ijsselhof R, et al. Mid-term outcomes in unbalanced complete atrioventricular septal defect: Role of biventricular conversion from single-ventricle palliation. European Journal of Cardio-Thoracic Surgery. 2017;**52**:565-572

[40] Buratto E, Ye XT, King G, et al. Long-term outcomes of single-ventricle palliation for unbalanced atrioventricular septal defects: Fontan survivors do better than previously thought. The Journal of Thoracic and Cardiovascular Surgery. 2017;**153**:430-438

[41] Owens GE, Gomez-Fifer C, Gelehrter S, Owens ST. Outcomes for patients with unbalanced atrioventricular septal defects. Pediatric Cardiology. 2009;**30**:431-435

[42] De Oliveira NC, Sittiwangkul R, McCrindle BW, et al. Biventricular repair in children with atrioventricular septal defects and a small right ventricle: Anatomic and surgical considerations. The Journal of Thoracic and Cardiovascular Surgery. 2005;**130**: 250-257. Erratum in: The Journal of Thoracic Cardiovascular Surgery. 2005;130:1195

[43] Delmo-Walter EM, Ewert P, Hetzer R, et al. Biventricular repair in children with complete atrioventricular septal defect and a small left ventricle. European Journal of Cardio-Thoracic Surgery. 2008;**33**:40-47

[44] Emani SM, McElhinney DB, Tworetzky W, et al. Staged left ventricular recruitment after single ventricle palliation in patients with borderline left heart hypoplasia. Journal of the American College of Cardiology. 2012;**60**:1966-1974

[45] Overman DM, Dummer KB, Moga FX, Gremmels DB. Unbalanced atrioventricular septal defect: Defining the limits of biventricular repair. Seminars in Thoracic and Cardiovascular Surgery: Pediatric Cardiac Surgery Annual. 2013;**16**:32-36

[46] Nathan M, Liu H, Pigula FA, et al. Biventricular conversion after single-ventricle palliation in unbalanced atrioventricular canal defects. The Annals of Thoracic Surgery. 2013;**95**:2086-2095

[47] Kalish BT, Banka P, Lafranchi T, et al. Biventricular conversion after single ventricle palliation in patients with small left heart structures: Short-term outcomes. The Annals of Thoracic Surgery. 2013;**96**:1406-1412

[48] Bailey L, Concepcion W, Shattuk H, et al. Method of heart transplantation for treatment of hypoplastic left heart syndrome. The Journal of Thoracic and Cardiovascular Surgery. 1986;**92**:1-9

[49] Rao PS, Covitz W, Moore HV. Principles of palliative management of patients with tricuspid atresia. In: Rao PS, editor. Tricuspid Atresia. Mount Kisco, NY: Futura Publishing Co.; 1982. pp. 233-253

[50] Rao PS, Covitz W, Chopra PS. Principles of palliative management of patients with tricuspid atresia. In: Rao PS, editor. Tricuspid Atresia. 2nd ed. Mt. Kisco, NY: Futura Publishing Co.; 1992. pp. 297-320

[51] de Leval M, McKay R, Jones M, et al. Modified Blalock-Taussig shunt: Use of subclavian orifice as a flow regulator in prosthetic systemic-pulmonary artery shunts. The Journal of Thoracic and Cardiovascular Surgery. 1981;**18**:112-119

[52] Gibbs JL, Orhan U, Blackburn MEC, et al. Fate of stented arterial duct. Circulation. 1999;**99**:2621-2625

[53] Siblini G, Rao PS, Singh GK, et al. Transcatheter management of neonates with pulmonary atresia and intact ventricular septum. Catheterization and Cardiovascular Diagnosis. 1997;**42**:395-402

[54] Alwi M, Choo KK, Latiff HA, et al. Initial results and medium-term follow-up of stent implantation of patent ductus arteriosus in duct-dependent pulmonary circulation. Journal of the American College of Cardiology. 2004;**44**:438-445

[55] Rao PS, Brais M. Balloon pulmonary valvuloplasty for congenital cyanotic heart defects. American Heart Journal. 1988;**115**:1105-1110

[56] Rao PS, Wilson AD, Thapar MK, Brais M. Balloon pulmonary valvuloplasty in the management of cyanotic congenital heart defects. Catheterization and Cardiovascular Diagnosis. 1992;**25**:16-24

[57] Rao PS. Pulmonary valve disease: Pulmonary valve in cyanotic heart defects with pulmonary oligemia. In: Sievert H, Qureshi SA, Wilson N, Hijazi Z, editors. Interventions in Structural, Valvular and Congenital Heart Disease. Boca Raton, FL: CRC Press; 2014. pp. 297-308

[58] Muller WH Jr, Danimann JF Jr. The treatment of certain congenital malformations of the heart by the creation of pulmonic stenosis to reduce pulmonary hypertension and excessive pulmonary blood flow; a preliminary report. Surgery, Gynecology & Obstetrics. 1952;**95**:213-219

[59] Rao PS. Pediatric hypoplastic left heart syndrome. Medscape Drugs & Diseases. 2016. Available from: http://emedicine.medscape.com/article/890196-overview

[60] Sano S, Ishino K, Kawada M, et al. Right ventricle-pulmonary artery shunt in first-stage palliation of hypoplastic left heart syndrome. The Journal of Thoracic and Cardiovascular Surgery. 2003;**126**:504-509

[61] Rao PS. Subaortic obstruction after pulmonary artery banding in patients with tricuspid atresia and double-inlet left ventricle and ventriculoarterial discordance (letter). Journal of the American College of Cardiology. 1991;**18**:1885-1886

[62] Rao PS. Further observations on the spontaneous closure of physiologically advantageous ventricular septal defects in tricuspid atresia with special emphasis on the surgical implications. The Annals of Thoracic Surgery. 1983;**35**:121-131

[63] Stansel HC Jr. A new operation for d-loop transposition of the great

vessels. The Annals of Thoracic Surgery. 1975;**19**:565-567

[64] Rao PS, Kulangara RJ, Moore HV, Strong WB. Syndrome of single ventricle without pulmonic stenosis but with left atrioventricular valve atresia and interatrial obstruction: Palliative management with simultaneous atrial septostomy and pulmonary artery banding. The Journal of Thoracic and Cardiovascular Surgery. 1981;**81**:127-130

[65] Jonas RA, Castaneda AR. Modified Fontan procedure: Atrial baffle and systemic venous to pulmonary artery anastomotic techniques. Journal of Cardiac Surgery. 1988;**3**:91-96

[66] Bartram U, Grunenfelder J, Van Praagh R. Causes of death after the modified Norwood procedure: A study of 122 postmortem cases. The Annals of Thoracic Surgery. 1997;**64**:1795-1802

[67] Tweddell JS, Hoffman GM, Mussatto KA, et al. Improved survival of patients undergoing palliation of hypoplastic left heart syndrome: Lessons learned from 115 consecutive patients. Circulation. 2002;**106**:82-89

[68] Yates MC, Rao PS. Pediatric cardiac emergencies. Emergency Medicine. 2013;**3**:164. DOI: 10.4172/2165-7548.1000164

[69] Tsounias E, Rao PS. Stent therapy for clotted Blalock-Taussig shunts. Congenital Cardiol Today. 2010;**8**(7):1-9

[70] Cashen K, Gupta P, Lieh-Lai M, Mastropietro C. Infants with single ventricle physiology in the emergency department: Are physicians prepared? The Journal of Pediatrics. 2011;**159**:273-277

[71] Schaff HV, Danielson GK. Corrective surgery for tricuspid atresia. In: Rao PS, editor. Tricuspid Atresia. Mount Kisco, NY: Futura Publishing Co.; 1982. pp. 275-292

[72] Freedom RM, Gow R, Caspi J, et al. The Fontan procedure for patients with tricuspid atresia: Longterm follow-up. In: Rao PS, editor. Tricuspid Atresia. 2nd ed. Mt. Kisco, NY: Futura Publishing Co.; 1992. pp. 377-386

[73] Kaulitz R, Ziemer G, Luhmer I, Kallfelz H. Modified Fontan operation in functionally univentricular hearts: Preoperative risk factors and intermediate results. The Journal of Thoracic and Cardiovascular Surgery. 1996;**112**:658-664

[74] Mosca RS, Kulik TJ, Goldberg CS, et al. Early results of the Fontan procedure in one hundred consecutive patients with hypoplastic left heart syndrome. The Journal of Thoracic and Cardiovascular Surgery. 2000;**199**:1110-1118

[75] Yoshimura N, Yamaguchi M, Oshima Y, et al. Risk factors influencing early and late mortality after total cavopulmonary connection. European Journal of Cardio-Thoracic Surgery. 2001;**20**:598-602

[76] Jacobs ML, Norwood WI Jr. Fontan operation: Influence of modifications on morbidity and mortality. The Annals of Thoracic Surgery. 1994;**58**:945-952

[77] Gentles TL, Mayer JE Jr, Gauvreau K, et al. Fontan operation in five hundred consecutive patients: Factors influencing early and late outcome. The Journal of Thoracic and Cardiovascular Surgery. 1997;**114**:376-391

[78] Gaynor JW, Bridges ND, Cohen MI, et al. Predictors of outcome after the Fontan operation: Is hypoplastic left heart syndrome still a risk factor? The Journal of Thoracic and Cardiovascular Surgery. 2001;**121**:28-41

[79] Stamm C, Friehs I, Mayer JE Jr, et al. Long-term results of the lateral tunnel Fontan operation. The Journal of

Thoracic and Cardiovascular Surgery. 2001;**121**:28-41

[80] Giannico S, Hammad F, Amodeo A, et al. Clinical outcome of 193 extra-cardiac Fontan patients: The first 15 years. Journal of the American College of Cardiology. 2006;**47**:2065-2073

[81] Azakie A, McCrindle BW, Van Arsdell G, Benson LN, Coles J, Hamilton R, et al. Extracardiac conduit versus lateral tunnel cavopulmonary connections at a single institution: Impact on outcomes. The Journal of Thoracic and Cardiovascular Surgery. 2001;**122**:1219-1228

[82] Kumar SP, Rubinstein CS, Simsic JM, Taylor AB, Saul JP, Bradley SM. Lateral tunnel versus extra-cardiac conduit Fontan procedure: a concurrent comparison. The Annals of Thoracic Surgery. 2003;**76**:1389-1396; discussion 1396-1397

[83] Kopf GS, Kleinman CS, Hijazi ZM, Fahey JT, Dewar ML, Hellenbrand WE. Fenestrated Fontan operation with delayed transcatheter closure of atrial septal defect. Improved results in high-risk patients. The Journal of Thoracic and Cardiovascular Surgery. 1992;**103**:1039-1047; discussion 1047-1048

[84] Fiore AC, Tan C, Armbrecht E, Huddleston CB, et al. Comparison of fenestrated and nonfenestrated patients undergoing extra-cardiac Fontan. The Annals of Thoracic Surgery. 2014;**97**:924-931; discussion 930-931

[85] Rao PS. Protein-losing enteropathy following the Fontan operation (editorial). The Journal of Invasive Cardiology. 2007;**19**:447-448

[86] Kannankeril PJ, Anderson ME, Rottman JN, Wathen MS, Fish FA. Frequency of late recurrence of intra-atrial reentry tachycardia after radiofrequency catheter ablation in patients with congenital heart disease. The American Journal of Cardiology. 2003;**92**:879-881

[87] Mavroudis C, Deal BJ, Backer CL. The beneficial effects of total cavopulmonary conversion and arrhythmia surgery for the failed Fontan. Seminars in Thoracic and Cardiovascular Surgery: Pediatric Cardiac Surgery Annual. 2002;**5**:12-24

[88] Rao PS. What an adult cardiologist should know about cyanotic congenital heart disease? Journal of Cardiovascular Diseases & Diagnosis. 2013;**1**:104. DOI: 10.4172/2329-9517.1000104

[89] Rao PS, Chandar JS, Sideris EB. Role of inverted buttoned device in transcatheter occlusion of atrial septal defect or patent foramen ovale with right-to-left shunting associated with complex congenital cardiac anomalies. The American Journal of Cardiology. 1997;**80**:914-921

[90] Hijazi ZM, Fahey JT, Kleinman CS, Kopf GS, Hellenbrand WE. Hemodynamic evaluation before and after closure of fenestrated Fontan. An acute study of changes in oxygen delivery. Circulation. 1992;**86**:196-202

[91] Balling G, Vogt M, Kaemmerer H, et al. Intracardiac thrombus formation after the Fontan operation. The Journal of Thoracic and Cardiovascular Surgery. 2000;**119**(4 Pt 1):745-752

[92] Varma C, Warr MR, Hendler AL, et al. Prevalence of "silent" pulmonary emboli in adults after the Fontan operation. Journal of the American College of Cardiology. 2003;**41**:2252-2258

[93] Monagle P, Cochrane A, Roberts R, et al. A multicenter, randomized trial comparing heparin/warfarin and acetylsalicylic acid as primary thromboprophylaxis for 2 years after the Fontan procedure in children. Journal

of the American College of Cardiology. 2011;**58**:645-651. DOI: 10.1016/j.jacc.2011.01.061

[94] Rao PS. Stents in the management of vascular obstructive lesions associated with congenital heart disease. In: Vijayalakshmi IB, editor. Cardiac Catheterization and Imaging (From Pediatrics to Geriatrics). New Delhi, India: Jaypee Publications; 2015. pp. 573-598

[95] Rao PS. Transcatheter embolization of unwanted blood vessels in children. In: Rao PS, Kern MJ, editors. Catheter Based Devices for Treatment of Noncoronary Cardiovascular Disease in Adults and Children. Philadelphia, PA: Lippincott, Williams & Wilkins; 2003. pp. 457-473

[96] Tsounias E, Rao PS. Versatility of amplatzer vascular plug in occlusion of different types of vascular channels. Catheterization and Cardiovascular Interventions. 2008;**71**(7):P38

[97] Feldt RH, Driscoll DJ, Offord KP, et al. Protein-losing enteropathy after the Fontan operation. The Journal of Thoracic and Cardiovascular Surgery. 1996;**112**:672-680

[98] Giannico S, Hammad F, Amodeo A, et al. Clinical outcome of 193 extracardiac Fontan patients: The first 15 years. Journal of the American College of Cardiology. 2006;**47**:2065-2073

[99] Chiu NT, Lee BF, Hwang SJ, et al. Protein-losing enteropathy: Diagnosis with (99m) Tc-labeled human serum albumin scintigraphy. Radiology. 2001;**219**:86-90

[100] Mertens L, Dumoulin M, Gewillig M. Effect of percutaneous fenestration of the atrial septum on protein-losing enteropathy after the Fontan operation. British Heart Journal. 1994;**72**:591-592

[101] Lemes V, Murphy AM, Osterman FA, et al. Fenestration of extracardiac Fontan and reversal of protein-losing enteropathy: Case report. Pediatric Cardiology. 1998;**19**:355-357

[102] Kreutzer J, Keane JF, Lock JE, et al. Conversion of modified Fontan procedure to lateral atrial tunnel cavopulmonary anastomosis. The Journal of Thoracic and Cardiovascular Surgery. 1996;**111**:1169-1176

[103] Marcelletti CF, Hanley FL, Mavroudis C, et al. Revision of previous Fontan connections to total extracardiac cavopulmonary anastomosis: A multicenter experience. The Journal of Thoracic and Cardiovascular Surgery. 2000;**119**:340-346

[104] Lopez JA. Transvenous right atrial and left ventricular pacing after the Fontan operation: Long-term hemodynamic and electrophysiologic benefit of early atrioventricular resynchronization. Texas Heart Institute Journal. 2007;**34**:98-101

[105] Estner HL, Kolb C, Schmitt C, et al. Long-term transvenous AV-sequential pacing in a failing atriopulmonary Fontan patient. International Journal of Cardiology. 2008;**127**:e93-e95

[106] Brancaccio G, Carotti A, D'Argenio P, et al. Protein-losing enteropathy after Fontan surgery: Resolution after cardiac transplantation. The Journal of Heart and Lung Transplantation. 2003;**22**:484-486

[107] Gamba A, Merlo M, Fiocchi R, et al. Heart transplantation in patients with previous Fontan operations. The Journal of Thoracic and Cardiovascular Surgery. 2004;**127**:555-562

[108] Jayakumar KA, Addonizio LJ, Kichuk-Chrisant MR, et al. Cardiac transplantation after the Fontan or Glenn procedure. Journal of the American College of Cardiology. 2004;**44**:2065-2072